DISEASES AND PARASITES OF SWINE

DISEASES AND PARASITES OF SWINE

Editor
Gove Hambidge

BIOTECH
2014
Biotech Books
Delhi - 110 035

Original Title: Livestock Yearbook of Agriculture, 1942

ISBN10 81-7622-086-8
ISBN13 978-81-7622-086-6

Published by : **BIOTECH BOOKS**
1123/74, Tri Nagar,
DELHI – 110 035
Phone: 27383999
e-mail: biotechbooks@yahoo.co.in

Showroom : 4762-63/23, Ansari Road, Darya Ganj,
NEW DELHI - 110 002
Phone: 23245578, 23244987

Laser Typesetting : **Classic Computer Services**
Delhi - 110 035

Printed at : **Chawla Offset Printers**
New Delhi – 110 052

PRINTED IN INDIA

CONTENTS

Introduction 1

1. **Hog Cholera** 21
   C.N. Mcbryde

2. **Swine Erysipelas** 37
   H.W. Schoening, G.G. Grey, O.I. Osteen

3. **Enteritis of Swine** 49
   C.N. Dale

4. **Swine Influenza** 59
   C.N. Dale

5. **Miscellaneous Diseases of Swine** 73
   G.T. Creech

6. **Brucellosis (Infectious Abortion) in Swine** 92
   Adolph Eichhorn

7. **Mange of Swine** 98
   Marion Imes

8. **Hog Lice** 107
   O.G. Babcock, E.C. Cushing

9. **Internal Parasites of Swine** 112
   L.A. Spindler

10. **Trichinosis** 167
    Benjamin Schwartz

11. **Salt Tolerance and Salt Poisoning of Swine** **187**
N.R. Ellis

12. **Nutritional Diseases of Swine** **196**
Louis L. Madsen

Index **219**

INTRODUCTION

Diseases of Swine

To picture what hog cholera has done to the swine population during the great outbreaks of the past; imagine that some virulent diseases were to wipe out 13 million or more people in the United States in a single year. As McBryde points out, up to 1914, when hog cholera began to be controlled, it costs swine growers an average of at least 20 million dollars every year.

The disease is highly infectious and contagious, appears suddenly, and usually runs an acute course, ending in death. The chief clinical symptoms are loss of appetite, fever, and great weakness; a post mortem examination generally shows striking changes in the lymph glands and other, characteristic tissue injuries. In the North, severe outbreaks are largely confined to the late summer and fall, but they may occur at any season in the South.

The disease is spread by the secretions and excretions of infected animals; carcasses are also a menace and should be promptly rendered, burned, or buried deeply and covered with quicklime. Studies indicate that houseflies and stableflies may be important factors in disseminating hog cholera widely and rapidly. Since infection may be spread even during the incubation period, before visible symptoms appear, McBryde advises that all new hogs brought to the warm should be segregated and kept under observation for a period of 2 weeks. He also strongly emphasizes good sanitation and proper feeding as preventive measures.

There is no known drug that will cure or prevent the disease. The first big forward step in combating it was the discovery that it is caused by a virus, not by a bacillus, as was formerly thought to be the case. Following this discovery, the Bureau of Animal Industry succeeded in developing a preventive serum early in the 1900's. Prepared from the blood of hyperimmunized–that is, highly immunized–hogs, this serum gives an immunity lasting several weeks. If a small amount of virus or virulent blood is injected at the same time as the serum, however, the animal develops its own antibodies capable of fighting the virus, and the immunity thus produced usually lasts throughout its lifetime.

Simultaneous inoculation is now the method generally used in immunizing swine herds. The one great disadvantage is that for 2 or 3 weeks after vaccination the animal may suffer a set-back, its general resistance may be lowered, and it may fall a prey to such complications as infection by other disease germs or by intestinal parasites. In spite of such "breaks," immunization has been a tremendous boon to producers; many now make it a regular practice to have each year's pig crop vaccinated while the animals are small. The serum is produced commercially, and all that is made in establishments doing an interstate business is produced under strict supervision by the Bureau of Animal Industry.

In an effort to overcome the drawback mentioned, research workers recently discovered that if a certain aniline dye, crystal violet, is added to the virus and the mixture is incubated, the virus is so weakened that it produces no bad effects and yet creates an immunity which apparently lasts up to marketing age at least. This method is now being extensively tested. Since there is a lag of 2 or 3 weeks after vaccination before active immunity is produced by the crystal-violet vaccine, it probably cannot entirely supplant the older method, but it promises to be both cheaper and safer in many instances.

Swine Erysipelas

Schoening, Grey, and Osteen point out that swine erysipelas in its acute form appears suddenly and can run quickly through a herd, killing many of the hogs and making the rest unprofitable for market. Some of the typical symptoms in an acute outbreak are a scaly eczema, dryness, and red discoloration of the skin, patches of which may slough off; loss of pieces of the ears and tail; enlarged and evidently painful joints; swellings on the legs, ears, snout, and elsewhere; reluctance to move unless forcibly roused; and a high temperature. The disease may also take a low-grade, chronic form, characterized perhaps by a stubborn eczema or by swollen joints; or apparently healthy animals may harbour the organism in the tonsils, the intestines, or elsewhere.

Sheep, cattle, horses, dogs, turkeys, chickens, and ducks are all susceptible to swine erysipelas, as are human beings; handlers of livestock and livestock products are frequently infected. Fish-handler's disease, so-called, is due to the swine erysipelas organism, which has been found on the skin of many salt-water fish. Recent studies show that a large percentage of cases of swine arthritis–which has become widespread in recent years–may be due to erysipelas; at any rate the organism was recovered from more than three-fourths of 572 enlarged joints collected in 16 States.

The organism that causes swine erysipelas is a bacillus, long known to produce serious outbreaks of the disease in Europe but not definitely found in this country until about 20 years ago. The bacillus can live for a long time and apparently even propagate in certain soils, though it is rather easily destroyed by heat and by disinfectants. In acute cases, it is found in the blood and excretions of sick animals, so that their surroundings become contaminated, but exactly how the disease passes from animal to animal is not yet known. Because of certain difficulties in diagnosis, much attention has been given recently to the development of a serum test, and one is now available that, within limits, has proved to be of value when properly handled.

Control measures at present are somewhat uncertain. Chronic cases should be removed from the herd. Pens can readily be cleaned and disinfected, but this gives no assurance that the organism will not continue to exist somewhere in the soil and cause an outbreak later on. There is an anti-swine-erysipelas serum which will produce an immunity lasting 2 or 3 weeks, but it is effective only when given very early in the acute stage of the disease. In Europe the disease is combated much as hog cholera is in this country, by the use of a hyperimmune serum and a live culture given simultaneously, but the fear has been that the general use of this method in the United States might actually spread the disease in cases of mistaken diagnosis. A carefully planned large-scale experiment with this method is now being carried on, however, in certain sections where the disease is especially serious.

It is very important, in actual or suspected outbreaks of swine erysipelas, to get in touch with State and local veterinary services.

Enteritis of Swine

The term "enteritis" means an inflammation of the intestines, and there are many kinds of enteritis of swine, says Dale.

Necrotic enteritis, sometimes called paratyphoid and other names, is an infectious disease caused by a micro-organism known as *Salmonella choleraesuis.* The symptoms of the disease, often fatal, include a rise in temperature, diminished appetite, diarrhoea, emaciation, weakness, and prostration. In the beginning stages, the malady is frequently mistaken for hog cholera, with very serious results; for hog cholera virus-serum inoculations may be given, and the virus and the *Salmonella* together make a deadly combination. Whenever necrotic enteritis could possibly be present in a herd, extreme precautions must be observed in hog cholera immunization.

There is no satisfactory cure for necrotic enteritis, but rigid sanitary measures such as those recommended for the control of roundworms will go a long way toward preventing it. When a vitamin deficiency is a complicating factor, as sometimes happens, the ration must be corrected.

Swine dysentery, also called black or bloody scours, and by other names, is another serious enteritis, responsible for much mortality among hogs. Acute and infectious, its outstanding symptom is a profuse bloody diarrhoea. This disease, too, is especially deadly in combination with hog cholera and demands extra precautions in cholera immunization. No specific cause has been determined, but, in general, infected animals are found to have been directly or indirectly in contact with sales barns or public stockyards; and the disease frequently occurs in hogs following cattle. There is no satisfactory cure. Preventive measures must include a broad programme of sanitation, separation of sick and healthy pigs, quarantine of newly purchased animals, and other measures. Both necrotic enteritis and dysentery call for the services of a veterinarian.

Young pigs are subject to an enteritis, called scours, which annually wipes out large numbers of them, especially during the first few days of life, and is responsible for much of the heavy loss–often 50 percent or more–that occurs on many farms. The trouble has been attributed to faulty nutrition (especially of the sows during the gestation period), poor housing, poor care, and lack of sanitation.

If this is true, it would seem that farmers who neglect to follow good swine-husbandry practices are responsible for waste that affects the public as well as themselves.

Swine Influenza

Caused by the combined action of a virus and a germ, swine influenza is an acute, infectious, and highly contagious disease which, once started, spreads rapidly through a herd. Apparently improper housing and undue exposure to cold and dampness are predisposing factors. Sick animals, which should be given good care, usually recover rapidly after 5 or 6 days, but complications may retard recovery and increase the mortality from the disease. No medicinal remedy is known, and no vaccine is available for general use.

Swine influenza was first definitely described in 1919. Subsequent research on it has been closely associated with research on human influenza and has contributed a great deal to our present understanding of the human disease. For this reason, Dale describes the progress of the work in some detail. Some of the outstanding discoveries include the following:

(1) Swine influenza was successfully transmitted to healthy animals by instilling infected mucus into the nose (nasal instillation).

(2) A micro-organism, *Hemophilus influenzae suis*, was isolated from experimental cases but, when used alone, failed to produce the disease.

(3) Filtered material (virus), when used alone, produced only a mild form of the disease.

(4) Virus and the organism together produced typical swine influenza.

(5) Serum from the blood of pigs that had recovered from swine influenza neutralized the virus, or made it harmless.

(6) Serum from swine that had recovered from the virus disease alone neutralized a mixture of the virus and the organism.

(7) Intramuscular injection of the virus alone immunized pigs against true swine influenza without producing the disease.

(8) Virus from human causes produced influenza in ferrets, and when they recovered they were immune to the same

strain of virus. Serum from ferrets that had recovered neutralized the human virus. Human serum neutralized the human virus.

(9) Swine virus produced disease in ferrets. Ferrets that recovered from swine influenza were immune to human influenza, but the reverse was not true.

(10) Both the human and the swine virus produced disease in mice, which have since been used to test blood serum for antibodies.

(11) In mice, different strains of human virus acted differently in producing immunity against swine influenza. Mice immunized against swine influenza were resistant only to certain strains of the human virus.

(12) Serum from animals exposed several times instead of only once to either human or swine virus contained antibodies against both viruses.

(13) Human virus produced a mild disease in young pigs. When the virus and the swine influenza organism were mixed, the disease was more severe, but it was not quite the same as true swine influenza. (The human virus has not yet actually been isolated from swine in the field).

(14) Lungworms were found to harbour the swine influenza virus and may act as reservoirs to carry it over from season to season. The infected worms did not produce the disease in swine except in late fall, winter, and spring.

(15) A mixture of swine virus and the hemorrhagic septicemia, organism instilled intranasally into swine produced a disease like swine influenza.

Miscellaneous Diseases of Swine

Creech discusses more than a dozen different diseases or injuries of swine that for the most part are not covered elsewhere in this volume.

Swine pox is caused by two types of virus, and the disease is spread by lice. It seldom attacks pigs over 6 months old. Poxlike eruptions on the skin, starting as small reddened areas and developing into characteristic blisters, are the chief symptom; in acute cases there may also be dullness, weakness, loss of appetite, chills, and fever. There is no known cure for the disease, which may be disastrous to sucklings, especially if there are complications with other diseases. Sick pigs should be isolated and well cared for, and the hog houses and equipment should be thoroughly cleaned and disinfected. The best preventive is to eradicate lice according to the directions given in the article on that subject.

Infectious arthritis (*joint ill*, or *navel ill*) is a usually fatal disease of newly farrowed pigs due to infection of the navel at the time of birth by one or more of several different germs. The infection eventually spreads to the joints, causing arthrities. Symptoms usually include marked weakness and rapid emaciation. Since there is no known cure, prevention is extremely important. It consists for the most part in proper handling at the time of birth, disinfection of the navel, and, above all, the provision of strictly sanitary farrowing quarters.

Necrotic rhinitis (*bull nose*, or *sniffles*) is an infectious disease caused by a tissue-destroying micro-organism, usually picked up from filthy surroundings and gaining entrance through injuries around the mouth or nose. (A similar or identical disease of suckling pigs is called necrotic stomatitis, or infectious sore mouth.) Sneezing, swelling of the face and nose, and eventually extensive destruction of tissues are characteristic symptoms. In advanced cases the animals should be destroyed, but in the early stages the removal of puslike material and treatment with tincture of iodine may be effective. Good sanitation is the best preventive.

Goiter (*hairless pigs*) is discussed in the article on nutritional diseases of swine. It is due to iodine deficiency and can be prevented by supplying iodine to the pregnant sow.

Paralysis of the hindquarters (*posterior paralysis*) is evidenced first by a wobbly or unsteady gait and finally by complete inability to stand on the hind feet and dragging of the headquarters. The condition may be due to anyone of several causes, including vitamin and mineral deficiencies and infectious diseases and parasites. In other words, the paralysis is a symptom, and the cause is often very hard to discover; hence treatment is usually unsatisfactory. Perhaps the best preventive is a good diet.

Pneumonia, the result of irritation of the lung tissues, may also be due to several causes–dust and other foreign materials, disease germs, internal parasites. It is a very common accompaniment of other diseases. Chills, fever, and difficult breathing are common symptoms. One of the most important points about pneumonia in swine is to make sure whether or not it is accompanied by some other and perhaps more serious disease. Sick animals should be well cared for and specially fed. The best general preventive is good sanitation and care. In particular, hogs should not be allowed to become chilled in severe weather.

Mastitis (*mammitis*, or *garget*) is an inflammation of the udder caused by infection with various micro-organisms, which may enter through injured tissues. A general disturbance of the system may follow the original condition. Treatment in acute cases consists of hot and cold applications, a purgative, cleansing of wounds or sores, surgery of abscesses. Tumors caused by the ray fungus, by tuberculosis germs, or by botryomyces require surgery by a veterinarian.

Skin diseases discussed by Creech include:

(1) Erythema

This is a diffuse reddening and itching which sometimes accompanies serious diseases and is sometimes due to external irritation. Proper sanitation, good feeding, and eradication of lice are the general preventives.

(2) Urticaria (nettle rash)

Equivalent to hives in human beings, this condition may be due to digestive disturbances or external irritation and filthy surroundings.

(3) Eczema

This eruptive skin inflammation may be caused by improper feeding, an insanitary environment, and irritation by lice; or it may accompany more serious diseases. Prevention, of course, is related to these causes.

(4) Sunburn

This affects light-coloured hogs and can be prevented by supplying shade.

(5) Freezing, or frostbite

Pigs farrowed in winter in the North and improperly housed may have their ears and tails frozen. Hogs in transit may also suffer frostbite.

In most of these cases of skin inflammation or injury, there are simple remedies, described by Creech, which will give relief.

Swine plague, or hemorrhagic septicemia, is an infectious disease caused by an organism known as *Pasteurella suiseptica.* In the United States it usually occurs as a complication with other diseases, particularly hog cholera, and chiefly affects the lungs, giving rise to pneumonia. Common symptoms include a high temperature, spasmodic cough, discharge of mucus, or mucus mixed with pus, from mouth and nose, loss of appetite, constipation, bloody diarrhoea, and prostration. Death usually follows. Diagnosis is difficult, and a veterinarian should be consulted because of the danger of complications. There is no cure. Preventive serums, aggressions, and bacterins may be used, but the best preventive is good sanitation and care.

Brucellosis (Infectious Abortion) of Swine

Recent surveys show that so far brucellosis in swine is much more limited in extent than brucellosis in cattle, but the disease is extremely important from a public health standpoint because:

(1) *Brucella suis,* the organism in hogs (discovered in 1914), causes a more severe type of undulant fever in human beings than does the Bang's disease organism of cattle;

(2) Half of the cases of human infection are due to the organism found in hogs;

(3) Human infection frequently occurs in swine-raising localities and in packing plants. Eichhorn concludes that definite, systematic measures to control or eradicate brucellosis of swine are amply justified.

The disease, which may cause sterility in boars as well as abortion in sows, is usually introduced into a herd of swine through the purchase of an infected animal. It spreads through contaminated feed and water and the eating of aborted fetuses and fetal membranes. Diagnosis is made by isolating the *Brucella* organism from infected animals, and also by a blood test, which, however, is not so reliable with swine as it is with cattle. Since there is no known cure for the disease, control measures are confined to prevention. Animals that react to the blood test should be eliminated, and subsequently the herd should be tested frequently until there is no positive or suspicious reaction. The sanitary measures recommended in the article on brucellosis of cattle should also be applied.

Mange of Swine

Common mange of hogs, which is widespread in the United States, stunts the growth of young animals, delays fattening, and causes some deaths, the total penalty probably being about $2 an animal in infected herds. In addition, mangy hogs are usually docked 50 cents to $1.50 a hundred weight at the market. The aggregate losses due to common mange are very great every year. They are also unnecessary, since the disease cap easily be eradicated; but as Imes points out, the methods used by many producers are not adequate.

The symptoms of common mange include itching, inflammation and swelling of the skin, the formation of vesicles that break and discharge serum, and eventually a thickening and folding of the skin. Final diagnosis must be based on actually finding the mites, which live in burrows in the skin.

Control measures include good sanitation and careful feeding, cleaning up infected premises and disinfecting them with a coal-tar-creosote preparation, and treating the whole herd if any of the animals become mangy. (Incidentally, the sarcoptic or common mange mite is transmissible to human beings; hence after handling mangy hogs, the operator should bathe and change clothing). Treatment consists in dipping the hogs in unprocessed crude oil, processed oils–of which crank-case drainings are probably the cheapest–or lime-sulfur dip. Imes describes the methods of applying the dips in considerable detail. If a commercial or home-made dipping vat is not used, oil may be floated on top of the water in a properly constructed hog wallow.

In addition to sarcoptic mange, hogs are subject to demodectic mange, caused by a different mite. This disease spreads much more slowly in the herd than common mange, and it cannot be cured except at an unjustifiable expense. Hence any animal found to be affected by demodectic mange should be promptly disposed of or killed, the premises should be. disinfected, and the rest of the herd should be dipped as a precautionary measure.

Hog Lice

The female hog louse lays her eggs on hog bristles, chiefly back of the ears and around the shoulders, neck, and flanks. She also travels along a bristle to get to another hog in contact with her original host. The hog louse is large–about a quarter of an inch long–and it makes a fresh puncture in the skin every time it feeds. The punctures often become raw spots that serve as centers of infection by other parasites, and constant irritation by lice puts the hogs off feed and makes them lose condition. For both financial and humanitarian reasons, then, these insects should be controlled.

The methods of control, described by Babcockand Cushing, are easy and inexpensive.

(1) Use crude petroleum–either natural or processed crude oil–in a dipping vat or a simple concrete hog wallow, such as is used for mange. If a heavy processed oil is used, dilute it with not over 20 percent of distillate oil.

(2) If there are too few hogs to justify a dip or vat apply the crude oil by hand with a brush, mop, or cloth.

(3) Or apply kerosene emulsion by hand (not in a vat or wallow). To make the emulsion, dissolve ½ pound of soap in 1 gallon of warm water. Add 2 gallons of kerosene, mixing thoroughly to form an emulsion. Dilute this with 11 gallons of soft water. In all hand applications, distribute the insecticide evenly over the head and body, paying special attention to the armpits and the inside of the ears.

Keep freshly oiled hogs quiet and in the shade for at least 48 hours. Do not expose them to direct sunlight or allow them to become chilled or force them to move rapidly.

Internal Parasites of Swine

As in the case of all livestock, internal parasites are a constant drain on the vitality of swine and hence a menace to full production as well as to the profits of the producer. In addition to causing death and general unthriftiness, Spindler points out, they are responsible for a rather extensive condemnation of parts of carcasses in packing houses. There are two methods of combating them–treatment with worm medicines, and the use of carefully worked out management practices to prevent infection. In the case of swine (not necessarily of other animals), the second is by far the more important and effective. Like a military campaign, it must be based on a knowledge of the activities and the weak points of the enemy, hence the importance of scientific studies of the life histories of parasites.

Spindler first discusses the three great groups of worm parasites–tapeworms, flukes, and roundworms.

The tapeworms occur in swine only in the larval, not the adult stages. These larvae resemble swollen bladders; hence they are called bladder worms. Three kinds are important:

(1) The pork bladder worm, which invades the muscles and may occur in nerve tissues of swine, is the larva of a tapeworm that infects human beings. The latter excrete the worm eggs, which are then picked up by swine. Only a very small percentage of pigs are infected in the United States.

(2) The hydatid is the larva of a tapeworm that infests dogs and wolves. These animals pass the eggs, which are then picked up by swine. The chief point of attack in swine is the liver; other internal organs may also be involved. Human beings can also be infected by these worms in the larval stage.

(3) The thin-necked bladder worm is the larva of a tapeworm of dogs. It attacks the liver and abdominal organs of swine and may be fatal to young pigs.

The lung flukes and the liver flukes are more important as enemies of other animals than of swine.

Roundworms are the largest and most important group of worms infesting swine. Spindler discusses 10 different kinds.

(1) The gullet worm, which attacks the gullet and tongue, lives part of its life in certain dung beetles and cockroaches, which pick up the eggs from manure. Swine, in turn, eat the infected insects. Human beings can also be infected with these or similar worms.

(2) Two species of thick stomach worms are very important parasites of swine. They live part of their lives in dung beetles, and under certain conditions one of them can also be transmitted to swine through birds, snakes, and other reptiles. The red stomach worm does not live in an intermediate host but infests the soil directly from contaminated swine droppings.

(3) Intestinal threadworms also are picked up directly from contaminated soil. The larvae penetrate the skin or are swallowed, get into the blood stream, reach the lungs and then the throat, are swallowed again, and finally pass to

the small intestine. In a larval stage, these worms can penetrate the skill of human beings.

(4) Four species of nodular worms, the commonest worm parasites of swine in some sections of the United States, attack the blind gut and large intestine, where they produce lumps, or nodules, in which the young worms live for a time. The infective larvae are picked up directly from soil contaminated by droppings.

(5) Whipworms inhabit the blind gut and large intestine, and the eggs are picked up directly from soil infected by droppings.

(6) Lungworms are widespread parasites of swine, do great damage to young pigs, and may help to spread swine influenza. They live part of their lives in various species of earthworms, which pick up the eggs from swine droppings. Then pigs eat the earthworms.

(7) The kidney worm causes heavy losses in the South and may now be spreading northward. These worms become embedded in the kidneys and ureters, sometimes after considerable migrating in the body, and immense numbers of eggs are passed in the urine of infected swine. The larvae are picked up by the pigs from contaminated soil, and under certain conditions they can also penetrate the skin. The growth of infested animals is often markedly stunted.

(8) The hookworm, which infests the small intestine and may cause hemorrhages, is picked up in a larval stage from contaminated soil.

(9) Thorn-headed worms, which may reach a length of 12 inches or more, attach themselves to the wall of the small intestine by means of spines on the head. Eggs are passed in the droppings of swine and picked up by white grubs (insect larvae), which in turn are eaten by swine.

(10) Ascarids, or large intestinal roundworms, are very common and widespread swine parasites. They wander extensively in the body but tend to become localized as adults in the small intestine. A full-grown female may contain more than 25 million eggs, which are passed in huge numbers in the droppings of infected swine; the eggs are sticky enough to adhere wherever they fall. Even light infections can stunt animals; heavy infections can kill them.

So much for the worm parasites. Spindler also discusses four kinds of protozoa that are parasites of swine, though less is known about them than about the worms. Of these, (1) the amoebae parasitize the intestine and are said to cause dysentery and other disorders, just as similar protozoa do in human beings. (2) The balantidia probably have the same effect. (3) Coccidia invade the intestinal lining and produce an extensive destruction of tissues. (4) The *Sarcocystis* is common in garbage-fed hogs, invading the muscles and producing cysts which may appear as white specks.

Spindler points out that only three kinds of swine parasites can really be effectively removed by worm medicines–ascarids, nodular worms, and stomach worms; but it is worth while to treat swine for these worms. The treatment should be carried out by a veterinarian. The drugs chiefly used are chenopodium, santonin, hexylresorcinol, phenothiazine, and carbon disulfide. Removal of worms; of course, is no insurance against reinfection.

Two plans for swine management to avoid infection by parasites are discussed in considerable detail. The object of both is to break the life cycle of the parasites at its weakest point, the stage outside the host animal, and to build up the resistance of the animals by good nutrition.

The McLean County system of sanitation was first tried out extensively in McLean County, Ill., about 20 years ago. Essentially, it consists of the following procedures, each of which is the result of careful experimenting and should be carefully followed:

(1) Before the sows farrow, clean the farrowing pens thoroughly and scrub them with scalding water and lye. Then close them until farrowing time and allow no one to enter. Shut off any outside pens with dirt floors so they cannot be used by the pigs.

(2) Clean the sows with soap and water just before they are placed in the farrowing pens. After farrowing do not allow the sows or pigs out of the pens. Keep the pens clean and sanitary.

(3) Haul–do not drive–the pigs to a clean pasture. A stoneboat and crates may be used.

(4) Keep the young pigs in a clean pasture until they are at least 4 months old. This should not be a permanent pasture but one that has been cultivated and sown to a forage crop.

In the pasture provide an individual shelter house for each sow and her litter. Allow no other hogs to get into the pasture and do not let the pigs out.

Careful records of the results of following this system show that it affords about 98 percent protection against parasitic and associated diseases, reduces the loss of pigs to about 24 percent instead of the 50 percent usual under a nonsanitary system, and permits the marketing of pigs as much as 7 weeks earlier.

The second system was devised to meet the special needs of producers in the Southeast, where kidney worms are a major hazard, and it is based on a close study of the habits of this parasite. It involves the following steps:

(1) Shortly before farrowing, put the sows in a specially prepared pasture, plowed and seeded after it was last used by hogs.

(2) In sowing, leave a bare strip at least 5 feet wide on three sides of the pasture and 30 feet wide on the fourth side. On this wide bare strip place the farrowing or shelter houses, water barrel, creep for pigs, and feeding pen for sows.

(3) Keep the bare strip on all four sides free of all trash, litter, and vegetation, cultivating it from time to time if necessary.

(4) Place the creep for pigs and the feeding pen for sows some distance apart on the wide bare area and arrange the sow feeding pen so that the pigs cannot have access to it.

(5) Arrange the water barrel so that it cannot overflow and wet the soil.

(6) Place the farrowing houses–one for each sow–on the wide bare area some distance apart, about 6 feet from the fence and facing it. Allow no trash or litter to accumulate around them.

Spindler shows the part played by each of these steps in kidney, worm control. Analysis shows that the system results in the raising of more pigs, better and more economical gains, a saving of 3 weeks or more in time of marketing, larger dressing percentages, and the passing, by inspectors, of nearly all livers and kidneys for food in contrast with the condemnation of about 92 percent of the livers and 100 percent of the kidneys in hogs raised without any attempt to prevent infection by parasites.

Under both these systems good feeding is essential in addition to the sanitary practices outlined.

Trichinosis

Trichinosis is a serious disease of human beings acquired by eating raw or partially cooked pork infested with trichinae. The minute immature forms of these roundworms are carried by the lymph and the blood stream from the intestines to all parts of the body, finally settling down chiefly in the muscles, where they become enclosed in small, hard cysts. About 5 percent of the human cases are fatal. The symptoms are so easily confused with those of other diseases that mistaken diagnoses have been common, and supposed cases of typhoid, undulant fever, influenza, nephritis, tuberculous meningitis, gastroenteritis, colitis, rheumatic endocarditis, syphilis, and tuberculosis have turned out to be trichinosis. Recent investigations have shown that there is a high percentage of infection in the urban population of the United States–from 14 to 27 percent in unselected post mortem examinations; but only a small proportion of these are severe enough to produce any symptoms of trichinosis.

The disease is obviously important from a public health standpoint, and that is the angle from which Schwartz considers it. He tells how trichinae were first discovered in human muscles when an English medical student in 1835 came on small gritty particles that dulled his scalpel while he was dissecting; how an American scientist in 1846 found trichinae in pork he was eating; and how three German scientists in 1860 discovered that a woman who had supposedly died of typhoid had really died of trichinosis acquired from uncooked sausage. These were three of the steps that gradually disclosed the nature of the disease. During the investigations that followed it was found that a considerable number of animals, including rats and mice, harbour the parasites; cases of human trichinosis have been traced to the eating of the improperly cooked meat of bears and other animals.

As a safeguard against trichinosis, some countries require that samples of pork be examined microscopically for trichinae at the packing plant. Schwartz shows that this method is very uncertain of results as well as being expensive; sometimes infected pork has to be examined 20 or 30 times before the trichinae are discovered, and one study made over a long period of years showed that about a third of more than 6,000 cases of human trichinosis resulted from eating pork that had been inspected microscopically and passed as trichina-free.

To determine what percentage of hogs in the United States are infected, a much more accurate test has been developed. This consists in digesting the diaphragms of hogs in artificial gastric juice in an incubator and counting the number of trichinae remaining in the digestive juice. By this method, tests were made with large numbers of hogs, beginning in 1933. Of the farm-raised hogs, less than 1 percent were found to be infected, and about two-thirds of these contained the parasites in very small numbers. Of the garbage-fed hogs (which presumably had access to scraps of fresh pork) well over 6 percent were found to be infected, and in two-thirds of these the infections were more or less extensive. But among hogs fed cooked garbage, about one-half of 1 percent were found to be infected, and these only slightly.

Schwartz's conclusions:

There is no known practical method of inspecting hogs for trichinae.

Under Federal meat-inspection requirements, all pork in meat products intended to be used without cooking, or the products themselves, must be so treated by heating, special refrigeration, or special processing that any trichinae they might contain are killed. Only about 60 percent of the hogs consumed in this country are slaughtered in federally inspected plants.

All fresh pork and ordinary cured pork not specially prepared in this way under the eyes of trained inspectors should be thoroughly cooked. Proper cooking makes the pork absolutely safe.

In the case of garbage–fed hogs, garbage–or at least all pork scraps in it–should be sterilized by heat before being fed. This might be accomplished by voluntary action or through State and municipal laws.

To safeguard hogs on the farm from getting trichinosis, the farmer should not feed offal or any scraps containing raw pork, should not throw dead rats and mice into hogpens, and should burn or bury deeply in quicklime the carcasses of hogs and other animals that have died.

Salt Tolerance and Salt Poisoning of Swine

The amount of salt required by hogs is known to be small as compared with the amounts required by other livestock, but evidence regarding the amounts that are actually poisonous to the animals has been somewhat conflicting. Ellis undertakes to review the scattered work that has been done in this field and gives the hitherto unpublished results of recent experiments at the Beltsville Research Center, Beltsville, Md. In the Beltsville work some of the pigs received relatively enormous quantities of salt–in one case, as much as 20 percent of the ration for a period of 4 weeks–yet there was only one instance, an animal fed salt at a level of 8 percent of the ration, in which there were apparent signs of severe poisoning, beginning on the eighty, sixth day of the experiment. Nor did pigs starved for salt for a preliminary period suffer any ill effects when they were later given free access to salt.

There is very little danger, Ellis concludes, that the use of the animal protein supplements and mineral mixtures ordinary led in this country will lead to salt hunger. On the other hand, it does not seem likely, from the evidence he presents, that even relatively large amounts of sodium chloride, per se, will poison hogs. The danger seems to lie in giving pigs waste salt products such as old pickling brine or salt contaminated with other substances; these other substances in the brine or dry mixture may be severely poisonous.

Nutritional Diseases of Swine

As Madsen points out, nutritional diseases of swine can make economical production impossible and cause considerable mortality. Controlling these diseases is one of the first essentials of successful swine husbandry.

The protein concentrates ordinarily fed to hogs are good sources of phosphorus but not of calcium, which may be deficient in the ration. When the animals are confined indoors and fed largely on grains, without good sun-cured roughage and with no access to sunlight, they may also be short of vitamin D. The result is likely to be rickets, a bone disease that weakens the young pigs and possibly makes them susceptible to other diseases. Sunlight and high-grade sun-cured legume hay are the best sources of vitamin D, but in the North in winter it may be advisable also to use some such source as fish oil. Several feeds, listed by Madsen, are good sources of calcium.

The author suggests four different mineral mixtures that may be used as supplements with different kinds of rations.

An abundant supply of calcium is especially necessary for breeding animals. When brood sows are deficient in calcium, farrowing is difficult, the milk supply is low, and the few pigs that survive at weaning time are likely to be weak and unthrifty. Though a phosphorus deficiency is not very common in swine, it may occur when they are grazed on pasture or cultivated root crops, with little or no grain or suitable supplements.

One of the chief causes of unthriftiness and death among young swine, especially those farrowed in late fall, winter, or early spring and kept confined without access to soil or vegetation, is nutritional anemia, resulting from a lack of iron and copper. Young pigs need a regular supply of these minerals beginning shortly after birth. It may be furnished in various ways, including drenching the pigs or swabbing the udder of the sow with a mineral solution.

Iodine deficiency is discussed in Nutritional Diseases of Farm Animals.

A lameness like that of rickets but apparently due to a manganese deficiency has occurred in pigs fed certain rations. Wheat and oats are usually higher in this mineral than is corn.

Like other animals, swine are subject to fluorine poisoning, and they are apparently even more susceptible to selenium poisoning than are horses and cattle.

Vitamin A deficiency occurs most commonly in swine fed in the dry lot without sufficient feeds that are good sources of this vitamin. The serious results of such a deficiency include irregularity in breeding behaviour, abortion, the birth of dead or weak pigs, and failure in lactation. It is extremely important to feed sows and young growing swine rations that will enable them to store up reserves of vitamin A. Madsen discusses the feeds that are especially good sources.

Among the various B vitamins, a deficiency of thiamin has been produced only experimentally; though the requirement for reproduction and lactation is high, the vitamin is not likely to be deficient on a ration including plenty of whole cereal grains or pasture and well-cured legume forage. A deficiency of riboflavin, resulting in severe symptoms, has also been produced experimentally; skim milk, buttermilk, and whey are high in this vitamin, and yellow corn is a fair source. Nicotinic acid deficiency, according to recent experimental work, may be a factor in susceptibility to necrotic enteritis, which causes widespread losses among swine; further investigations are needed on this point. A deficiency of pyridoxine (vitamin B_6) has produced epileptic fits and a certain type of anemia in swine, according to recent experiments, but the vitamin is not likely to be lacking in ordinary swine rations. Pantothenic acid deficiency has been found to produce a degeneration of the sheath of the nerve fibers in young swine, resulting in muscular incoordination. A similar disorder that occurs in swine under farm conditions is of considerable economic importance, and experiments indicate that pantothenic acid deficiency is perhaps the chief cause. Dry heat treatment of swine feeds apparently destroys the vitamin, and in addition many common feeds apparently contain insufficient amounts.

Madsen discusses a highly fatal disease of newborn pigs apparently due to a marked lowering of blood sugar, which in turn is probably caused by failure to get enough food during the first few days after birth. Affected pigs can usually be saved in the early stages by injections of glucose and hand feeding. Suggested preventive measures include liberal feeding of sows and gilts throughout pregnancy and close watching of newborn pigs to make sure they get enough food and do not become chilled.

Chapter 1

HOG CHOLERA

C.N. McBryde[1]

[1] *C.N. McBryde was in charge of the Field Station, Pathological Division, Ames, Iowa, Bureau of Animal Industry, until March 1, 1942, when he retired.*

In its effects on swine, hog cholera can be compared only with some of the diseases that used to wipe out whole communities of human beings before the days of modern medicine. The discovery of a serum that would produce immunity against this disease was an event of major importance to the livestock industry. Here a pioneer in the fight against hog cholera tells what it is and what can be done about it.

Hog cholera is a devastating livestock disease that has caused enormous economic losses in the United States for over a century. It recurs from year to year but during certain periods has been unusually prevalent. The first such period on record reached its climax in 1887, the second in 1896, and a third in 1913. During these periods hog producers suffered enormous losses, and in some localities the swine population was almost wiped out. In the fall of 1926 the disease again became unusually prevalent in parts of the Middle West. The supply of preventive serum on hand at that time was inadequate to meet the unusual demand, and losses in some sections were very heavy.

The direct monetary value of hogs destroyed by cholera in the United States has amounted to as much as 65 million dollars in a single year, and the average annual loss during any 10-year period prior to 1914 was probably not less than 20 million dollars. If the indirect losses could be computed, the totals would be greatly increased.

The estimated numbers of hogs dying from cholera is the United States from 1884 to 1940 inclusive are shown in Fig. 1. According to data available, the disease killed more than 13 percent of the swine in the country in 1896. Again in 1913 more than 10 percent of the hogs in the United States died of cholera. Since 1914, except for 1926, as noted previously, the general trend of losses from hog cholera has been downward as a result of the increasing use of anti-hog-cholera serum.

It does not appear to be definitely established whether hog cholera originated in America or in Europe. According to some authorities the disease existed in Europe long before it was recognized in this country, and it seems not unlikely that the contagion may have been imported from there, as was pleuropneumonia of cattle. It was first reported in the United States in southern Ohio in 1833 and soon spread throughout the country. By 1853 no less than 90 separate areas of infection were known to exist, and the malady was becoming much dreaded by swine breeders. Hog cholera now occurs in every State in the Union and in practically all parts of the world where hogs are raised. In Canada and Australia, however, the losses from the disease are said to be comparatively small in proportion to the number of pigs raised.

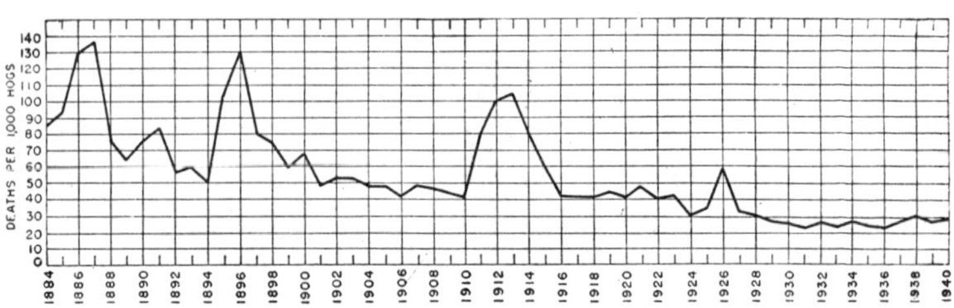

Fig. 1: Estimated death losses of hogs from hog cholera in the United States 1884-1940.

The Cause of Hog Cholera

Hog cholera has been under investigation by the United States Department of Agriculture since 1878. Because of its very great importance to the livestock industry it was one of the first diseases to be studied experimentally by the Bureau of Animal Industry after its establishment in 1884.

As a result of early studies carried out in the laboratories of the Bureau of Animal Industry of the United States Department of Agriculture, it seemed to be definitely established in 1885 that a bacterium, or bacillus, resembling the germ that causes typhoid fever in man, was the cause of hog cholera. For nearly 20 years this germ, which came to be called the hog cholera bacillus, was quite generally accepted by research workers in the field of animal diseases as the cause of hog cholera. Later studies by the Bureau of Animal Industry, however, proved that this germ is not the true cause of the disease and established the fact that it is caused by a virus.

The virus of hog cholera cannot be seen with the most powerful microscopes in use today, and it passes readily through the pores of very fine filters which hold back all visible bacteria. It is therefore called an ultramicroscopic virus and a filtrable virus. Attempts to grow the virus outside of the animal body generally have been unsuccessful. However, Carl Tenbroeck, director of the Department of Animal Pathology of the Rockefeller Institute, has recently reported that he has been able to grow the virus by methods similar to those previously described by Hecke, a German investigator.

The discovery that hog cholera is caused by a filtrable, ultramicroscopic virus was very important in the study of this disease. It upset all previous concepts regarding the nature of the disease and served to explain earlier failures to obtain an effective vaccine or serum. It also paved the way for subsequent studies that finally led to the discovery of a successful preventive serum.

Symptoms and Diagnosis

Hog cholera is a highly infectious and contagious disease. It affects swine of all ages and is usually acute, although it sometimes pursues a subacute or chronic course. It is characterized by a sudden onset, loss of appetite, fever, and weakness. The mortality rate of the acute form is usually high, and entire herds have been wiped out by it within a short time. Pigs affected with the disease in the subacute or chronic form may linger for some time before they succumb. Spontaneous recovery is rare.

All breeds of swine are subject to the disease. At one time it was thought that the mulefoot, or single-toed, hog was immune, but this was proved to be a fallacy by experimental inoculation of these animals.

When the disease makes its appearance in a herd, the first symptoms noted are loss of appetite in one or more animals, which either refuse to come up to feed with the rest of the herd or come to the feed trough, nibble at their feed, and then turn away. In animals experimentally infected, fever usually develops a day or two before visible symptoms are noted.

The affected animals separate themselves from the rest of the herd and soon show signs of weakness, especially in the hind legs, which are frequently crossed, resulting in a peculiar wobbling, scissors-like gait. The fever rises rapidly in the acute cases, and the animals may become very thirsty. Frequently there is a conjunctivitis, characterized by a thick, gummy secretion, which at times may almost glue the eyelids shut. The sick pigs usually die within 7 to 10 days.

In diagnosing hog cholera, the temperature of the affected animals is of much importance. The normal temperature of swine under ordinary weather conditions, when the animals are at rest and not excited, ranges from 101° to 103° F. When cholera is present in a herd, it is not uncommon to find a large proportion of the hogs with temperatures of 104° to 107° F., or even higher. The body temperature usually falls in the later stages of the disease and frequently becomes subnormal shortly before death.

A pig sick with hog cholera has a rather characteristic appearance. The animal stands in a listless, dejected attitude with the head drooping downward and the tail hanging straight and limp. As a field man of the Bureau of Animal Industry expressed it, the animal appears to be lost in thought (Fig. 2).

In most cases it is not possible to know when the infection actually reaches a farm herd, but once the disease makes its appearance it spreads more or less rapidly throughout the herd if no treatment is given. A large part of the herd does not sicken suddenly, however, as is the case in an outbreak of swine influenza, or "hog flu."

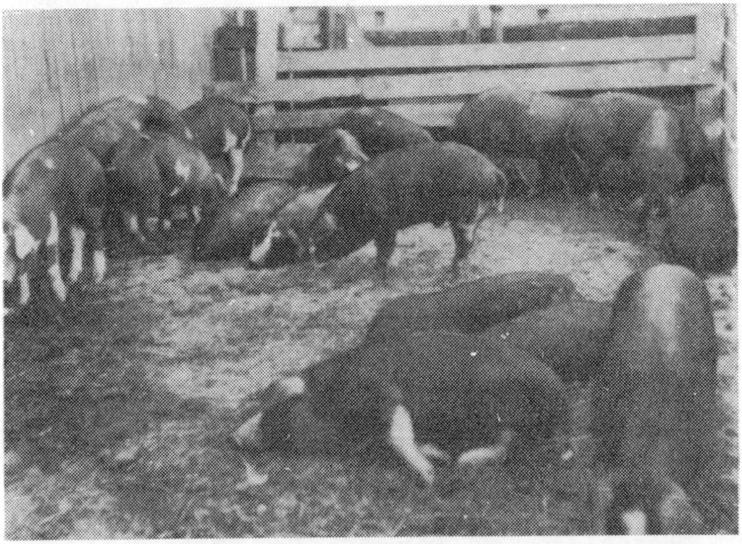

Fig. 2: Pigs suffering from acute hog cholera. The sickest animals are lying down; the others stand in the characteristic attitude, with heads down and tails limp.

In the course of virus production at the Bureau of Animal Industry station at Ames, Iowa, hog cholera virus was injected into the bodies of 100 susceptible shotes. The shortest incubation period (the time between the entrance of the virus into the body of the animal and the appearance of visible symptoms) was 3 days and the longest 5 days, the average being about 4 days. When susceptible swine are exposed by contact, it is impossible to determine just when infection takes place, but visible symptoms are rarely observed within less than 5 or 6 days after such exposure.

Seasonal Occurrence

Hog cholera has a rather marked seasonal incidence. In the Middle West it is essentially a disease of the late summer and fall, as shown in Fig. 3. During the winter months outbreaks are sporadic, and the disease never becomes epidemic as in the summer and fall. In the South, where the winters are mild and the temperature more or less uniform, severe outbreaks of hog cholera may occur at any season of the year.

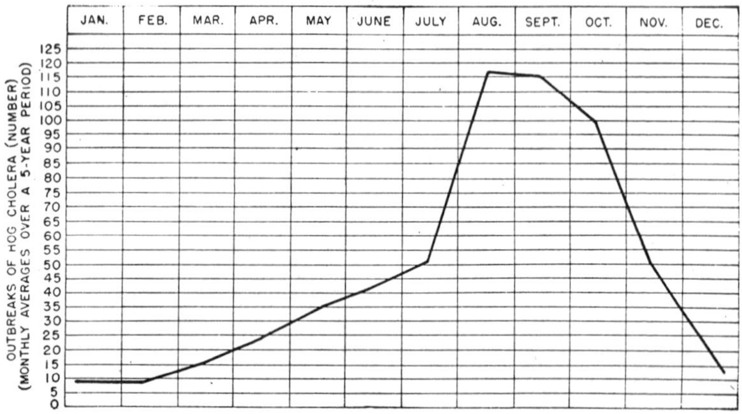

Fig. 3: Seasonal occurrence of hog cholera in Iowa, based on a 5-year record, 1928-32.

Before the discovery of a preventive serum, the disease often swept through the countryside, causing devastating losses. During the fall months, looking across the prairies of the Middle West, one could often see smoke ascending from perhaps half a dozen farms where pigs dead of cholera were being burned. The writer recalls such sights in 1904 to 1906, the early years of his field work with cholera in Iowa and Nebraska.

Post Mortem Findings

The skin of the under surface of the body and behind the ears is frequently bright red at the height of the disease and later may become dark purplish.

The changes that take place in the lymph glands of hogs with cholera are usually quite striking and are of considerable diagnostic importance. These glands are normally gray, but in hog cholera they become enlarged and show marked reddening. When the glands are cut through, it is often found that the reddening is confined to the margin and does not extend throughout the body of the gland. The lymph glands are quite generally affected. The ones usually found on post mortem examination to be diseased are those in the neck near the angle of the jaw, those in the groin, and those in the mesentery, or thin membrane which supports the intestines.

The lungs show small hemorrhagic spots on the outer surface, varying in size from that of bird shot to that of a small pea and usually bright red in colour. Another frequent lesion, or tissue injury, is caused by the collapse of lung lobules, giving rise to larger areas of a dark-red or purplish colour.

The spleen, or milt, is usually engorged with blood, darker than normal, and often soft and easily torn. Not infrequently dark, raised, ovoid areas a quarter of an inch or more long are seen along the border of the spleen.

The kidneys usually show characteristic, lesions in the form of small, more or less circular hemorrhages, varying from pin-point to pin-head size. These are perhaps the most characteristic of all lesions of hog cholera. They are shown in Fig. 4. They are best observed after the thin capsule surrounding the kidney has been stripped away. The hemorrhages may be few in number, but at other times the surface may be thickly studded with them, giving rise to the so-called turkey-egg kidney. The bladder usually shows small hemorrhages on the inner lining like those seen on the kidneys.

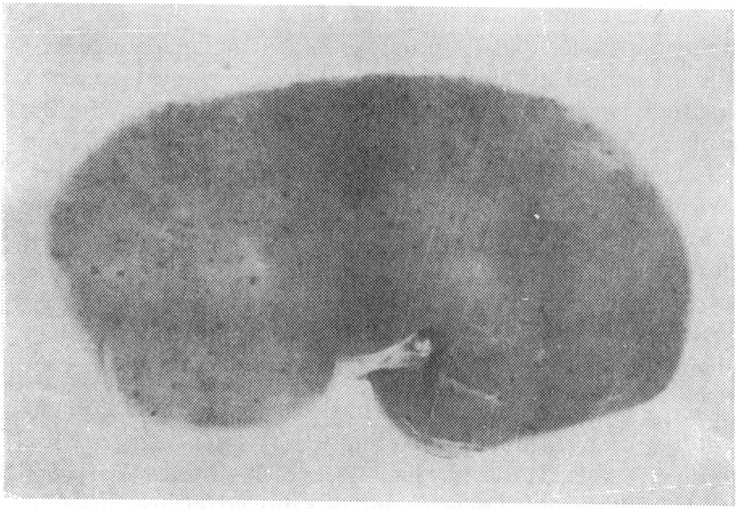

Fig. 4: Hog kidney showing lesions characteristic of acute hog cholera.

The intestines sometimes show small red hemorrhages on the outer surfaces and also on the inner lining. The lining of the upper part of the large intestine often shows a diffused reddening. In the subacute or chronic cases the lining of the large intestine often becomes ulcerated, and this is especially noticeable where the small intestine joins the large intestine. Distinct, raised ulcers may occur in the large intestine. When well-defined, these are called button ulcers.

Marked variation in the extent of the lesions is a peculiarity of the disease. At times they may be so slight as to be scarcely noticeable; again, they may be very extensive and very striking. Since tissues and organs of hogs dying from other causes may present an appearance very similar to that described for hogs dead of cholera, it is not advisable for a farmer to attempt to determine the cause of death by cutting open a dead hog. A veterinarian should always be called in when disease appears in a herd.

Modes of Infection

That the sick pig is a potent factor in the spread of hog cholera has long been known, but the manner in which the virus is thrown off from the animal body has not been so well understood. Experiments conducted at the Bureau field station at Ames, Iowa, have demonstrated that the virus is present in the circulating blood of the sick animal and also in the various secretions and excretions. It was found in the circulating blood of a sick pig as early as the first day after experimental infection. The virus was found in the eye and nose secretions and the fecal matter by the third day and in the urine by the fourth day. It is apparent that the cholera-infected pig may be a source of danger during the period of incubation, that is, before the development of visible symptoms of the disease. In purchasing new stock, therefore, the farmer should segregate, such animals and keep them under observation for at least 2 weeks before adding them to his herd.

At one time it was thought that birds, especially pigeons, might be an important factor in spreading the disease. Farmers were accordingly advised to destroy their flocks of these birds. That belief was purely theoretical, however, and was proved false by carefully conducted experiments in which susceptible pigs were exposed for long periods to pigeons which passed back and forth from a pen only 10 feet away that contained pigs sick and dying of hog cholera. Although pigeons were shown not to be concerned in the dissemination of hog cholera, it is not unlikely that crows and buzzards may act as carriers of the disease, for these birds may carry away and later drop portions of cholera-diseased carcasses upon which they have fed.

The virus has been found to remain active throughout the winter in the carcasses of cholera-infected pigs buried late in the fall in Iowa. Unburied carcasses of infected pigs were found to remain infectious for 11 weeks during cold weather. In earlier times such carcasses were undoubtedly a potential menace, but now-a-days dead animals on farms are usually picked up promptly by trucks operated by rendering plants. If such service is not available, all carcasses of hogs should be burned or else buried deeply and covered with quicklime. During the warm summer months, both buried and unburied carcasses undergo rapid putrefaction, and the virus is soon destroyed. In warm weather, after the virus leaves the animal body in the secretions and excretions, it is quickly inactivated, but in cold weather it may survive for a much longer time. Contaminated pens were found to harbour the infection for as long as 4 weeks during the winter season, whereas in summer they were sometimes no longer infectious after 24 hours. The rapid disappearance of the virus from contaminated pens in hot weather is probably a result of putrefactive and fermentative changes taking place in the litter. Sunlight is also potent in the destruction of disease organisms.

Cured meats are unquestionably a source of danger when fed as scraps in garbage, since the virus has been found to survive in hams taken from cholera-infected hogs cured by both the dry-salt and brine methods.

A study of insects as possible carriers of hog cholera was made some years ago at the field station at Ames. The species studied included the common hog louse, the housefly, the biting stablefly, the buffalo gnat, and several species of mosquitoes. Extensive experiments demonstrated quite conclusively that both the housefly and the stablefly were capable of transferring the virus of hog cholera from sick to well pigs. The results for the other insects were negative.

The housefly commonly feeds on the highly virulent eye secretions of hogs suffering from cholera as well as on the infectious blood from wounds or cuts. Since experiments by the United States

Bureau of Entomology and Plant Quarantine have demonstrated that houseflies can travel as far as 12 miles in 48 hours, it is plain that these flies may contribute to the rapid spread of hog cholera from farm to farm.

It was demonstrated that the virus of hog cholera may be transmitted from sick to well pigs through the bite of the stablefly. Not much is known as to the flight habit of stableflies except that they will follow a team of horses for a considerable distance along a highway. After engorging themselves with blood, they have a habit of resting for a while on the vegetation along the roadside and then following another team of horses. In such relays they may travel a considerable distance. In the late fall, too, the flies may enter the open windows of automobiles and thus be transported long distances. Weekly counts of flies trapped on dairy farms near Ames were made during the summer and early fall for several years. Curves or graphs plotted to show the prevalence of the biting flies were found to correspond very closely to those showing the incidence of hog cholera during the several years in which the fly counts were made. Insect transmission provides the most satisfactory explanation of the rapid spread of hog cholera during an outbreak and the fact that it frequently seems to jump from one farm to another, often skipping over intervening farms.

Importance of Sanitation and Care in the Prevention of Disease

Sanitation, proper feeding, and good care are of the greatest importance in successful swine raising.

A recent survey by an authority on swine diseases has revealed, however, that only about one-third of the farmers of this country follow good practices in feeding and housing their swine.

Poor feeding undoubtedly tends to lower the resistance of livestock to many infectious diseases. Recent experimental work indicates, for example, that a ration lacking in certain vitamins may be a hitherto unsuspected factor in certain intestinal troubles of swine. Poor housing is a predisposing factor in pneumonia, influenza, and other respiratory disturbances.

Sanitation is probably the most neglected factor in swine raising, and its lack undoubtedly contributes to the occurrence of fifth-borne intestinal diseases. The practice of using old hog lots year after year should be discontinued. When pigs are allowed to run in such lots they are almost certain to pick up the eggs of intestinal parasites and the germs of disease, and as a result the farmer will have a lot of unthrifty, unprofitable pigs on his hands.

Among the ailments of swine the intestinal diseases are next in importance to hog cholera. They not only cause an enormous direct loss but are also responsible for a large indirect loss. The simultaneous vaccination of such infected herds with serum and virus for immunization against hog cholera is likely to be followed by bad results.

In 1927 the Bureau of Animal Industry, through carefully conducted experiments carried out in McLean County, Ill., developed what has become known as the McLean County system of swine sanitation. While the system was developed primarily for the protection of swine against infestation with the ascaris, or common roundworm, it has also served to protect them against the filth-borne bacterial diseases. In this way it has proved a valuable adjunct in the successful immunization of swine against hog cholera.

Prevention of Hog Cholera

Many preparations composed of various drugs and chemicals have been exploited from time to time as preventives of or remedies for hog cholera, but all such products tested by Federal and State institutions have been found worthless. Farmers are therefore warned against investing their money in such preparations.

Many so-called tonics also are advertised as able to do wonders for hogs. Some of them may have some value as conditioners, but none are of any value in the prevention or cure of hog cholera.

Anti-Hog-Cholera Serum

After the discovery that hog cholera is caused by a filtrable, or ultramicroscopic, virus, a few preliminary experiments looking toward production of a protective serum were carried out in 1903 at the Bureau of Animal Industry experiment station at Bethesda, Md. Results were not satisfactory, and the experiments were laid aside on account of other work. In 1905 the experiments were resumed at the Bureau field station at Ames, Iowa. A successful preventive serum was finally developed there and was given a practical trial on farms in the vicinity of Ames in 1907.

The method of preparing the serum was patented, and all rights were dedicated to the public. Notice of the successful results was sent to every State, with an invitation to send representatives to the Bureau station at Ames to observe the methods of preparing and administering the serum. Twenty-five States accepted this invitation in 1908. During the years immediately following these demonstrations, a number of States began production and distribution of the new serum to farmers within their borders. At the same time or shortly after the preparation and sale of the serum were undertaken by commercial concerns, and when these firms became well established serum production by the States was discontinued.

The serum is prepared by injecting large immune hogs with virulent blood obtained from pigs sick of cholera. A very minute quantity of such blood would cause the death of a susceptible hog, but even large doses are harmless to an immune hog. After the immune hogs are injected with virulent blood they are called hyperimmunes, since their immunity is increased by this procedure. After a suitable interval, the hyperimmune hog is bled by cutting off a portion of its tail. Several bleedings are made in this manner. This blood contains large quantities of protective substances termed antibodies. Anti-hog-cholera serum is prepared by removing the fibrin and cells from the blood and adding a small amount of preservative to the clear serum.

The efficacy of anti-hog-cholera serum in the prevention of hog cholera is now universally recognized, and the serum is used in all parts of the world where hogs are raised. It is not a cure for hog cholera and should be used only as a preventive, although it seems to have some curative value if administered in the very early stages of the disease.

When given alone, the serum produces only a temporary immunity, which may be lost within a few weeks. When the serum is given in conjunction with a small amount of virus or virulent blood, however, a solid, or lasting, immunity is produced which usually persists throughout the lifetime of the animal. Because of the permanence of the immunity, this method of administering the serum, known as simultaneous inoculation, or serum-virus immunization, is generally employed in the immunization of herds of swine. The serum may be injected under the skin of the flank or in the axillary space between the foreleg and body. In small pigs some practitioners favour injecting the serum into the abdominal cavity of small pigs, while it may be injected behind the ear in large animals. The two methods most commonly employed in giving the serum and virus are shown in Figs. 5, *A* and *B*.

The dose of serum varies with the weight of the animal. The minimum doses prescribed by the Bureau of Animal Industry are shown on all commercial labels. If cholera has appeared in a herd before treatment is given, the amount of serum should be increased by half.

Because the dose increases with the weight of the animal, it is more economical to immunize swine against cholera when they are small. When pigs are left unvaccinated there is also additional risk of loss. Many farmers therefore make it a routine practice to have each year's crop of pigs immunized while young. Immunization at about weaning time is recommended.

Since an active virus is used in simultaneous, or serum-virus, immunization-commonly termed vaccination–it is of the utmost importance that the animals receiving this treatment be perfectly healthy and free from disease. After treatment, there is a period of lowered resistance in the animals, owing to the fact that the virus circulates in the blood for 2 or 3 weeks after vaccination. If the animals are perfectly healthy at the time of treatment, are not harbouring any infection and are not exposed to infection shortly after treatment, there is no danger connected with this method of immunization. If, however, the pigs happen to be harbouring a masked or unsuspected infection at the time of treatment or become exposed to infection shortly thereafter, trouble may develop, and so-called breaks may occur. Such unfortunate occurrences are really not breaks in immunity but result from the combined action of the virus, and some other infective agent. The period of lowered resistance which accompanies serum-virus treatment results from a decrease in the number of white blood cells, which are known to be one of the main defences of the animal body against infection. The decrease in white cells has been found to be less when large doses of serum are given, and therefore it is advisable to give ample doses of serum in carrying out the simultaneous, or serum-virus, treatment.

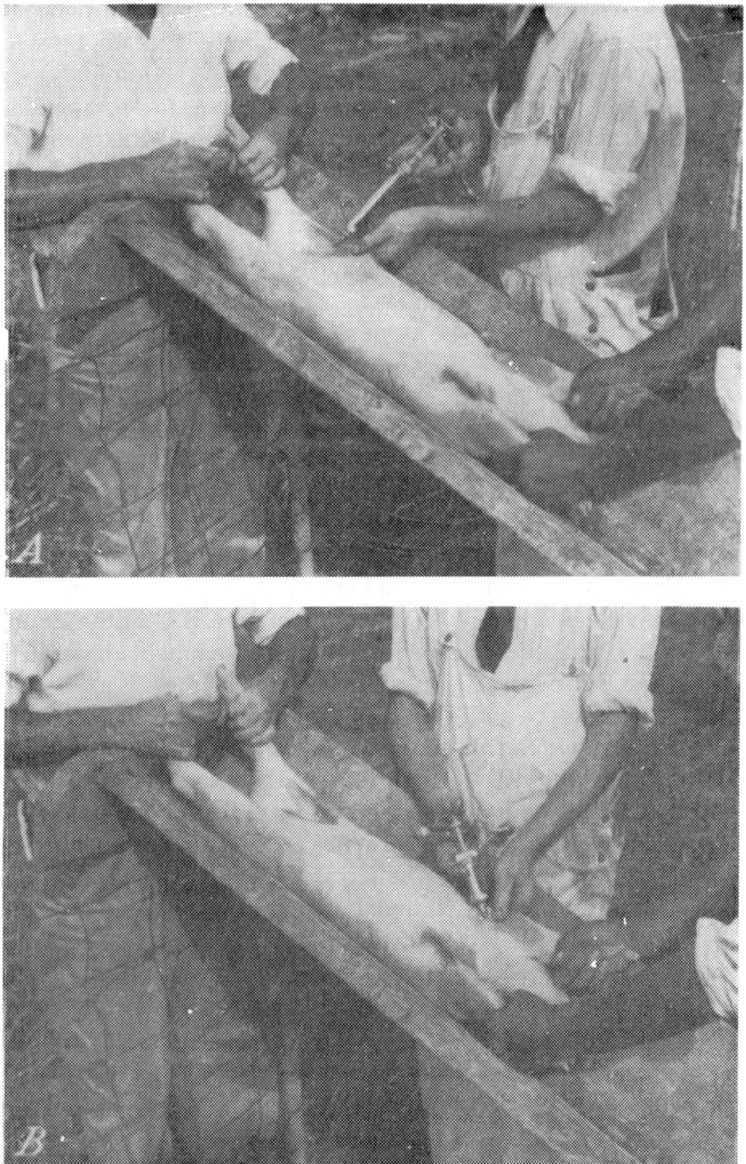

Fig. 5: *A*: Injecting a pig with anti-hog-cholera serum beneath the skin in the Flank. *B*: Injecting virus in the axillary space between the foreleg and the body.

Anti-hog-cholera serum is now produced on a large scale in the United States by many commercial plants throughout the country, the majority of which, however, are located in the hog-raising States of the Middle West, where suitable animals are readily obtainable. In 1913 Congress passed an act placing these plants under the supervision of the United States Bureau of Animal Industry. A new division was accordingly established, designed as the Division of Virus-Serum Control, which maintains a rigid supervision, through its trained veterinary and lay inspectors, of all commercial plants engaged in the production of anti-hog-cholera serum and hog cholera virus, as well as of other biological products intended for veterinary use. Before any anti-hog-cholera serum leaves a commercial plant, samples are subjected to rigid tests for potency, carried out under the supervision of Federal veterinary inspectors. Samples of all virus used with anti-hog-cholera serum are likewise tested. The swine raiser who has his pigs immunized against hog cholera is, therefore, sure of having standardized and reliable products used on his herd, provided the veterinarian who does the work has handled the products in a proper manner after receiving them from the producer.

Crystal-Violet Vaccine

Scientific workers in the Bureau of Animal Industry have sought for many years to develop a protective vaccine from which the disease-producing properties of the active virus would be completely eliminated.

Much time and work have been devoted to the preparation and testing of experimental vaccines at the station at Ames during the last 15 or 20 years. Various chemical agents have been used in the preparation of vaccines, and in some cases effective vaccines were obtained. The results were not uniform and consistent, however, until crystal violet, an aniline dye, was tried as an attenuating, or weakening, agent with a view to reducing virulence. It was found that the addition of this chemical to virus-infected blood entirely eliminated the disease-producing property of the virus without affecting its antigenic, or immunizing, property.

The new immunizing agent so developed was subjected to carefully controlled experimental tests at the Bureau field station and has been used successfully on more than 12,000 pigs in 236 farm herds in the vicinity of Ames. Pigs treated with this vaccine show no visible reaction, and there is no danger of introducing hog cholera on noninfected premises through its use. The absence of any reaction period following the administration of crystal-violet vaccine, with no apparent loss of appetite and no necessity for change of ration, provided a good one is being supplied, insures an uninterrupted gain in weight. In turn this should effect somewhat earlier marketing than is possible with pigs receiving serum-virus treatment, which usually necessitates a reduction in the feed for a time.

Although the duration of the immunity following treatment with crystal-violet vaccine has not been definitely established, it seems to protect swine against hog cholera satisfactorily through the fattening period or up to the usual market age, which is about 8 months in Iowa. Unfortunately there is an interval of 2 or 3 weeks between the administration of the vaccine and complete establishment of immunity, and this will naturally limit its use to some extent in veterinary practice, for it could not be used in a community where hog cholera is prevalent. For the same reason, the vaccine could not be used on garbage-feeding ranches where the pigs are farrowed on the ranch. It might be used, however, on garbage-feeding ranches which bring in pigs from the outside if the pigs receiving the vaccine are held in quarantine for 3 weeks and fed on grain before being put on the garbage ration. The vaccine cannot, therefore, entirely supplant the serum-virus method of immunization, but it may find a field of usefulness in the treatment of farm herds in the spring and early summer before hog cholera becomes prevalent. It should also afford a somewhat cheaper and safer means of protection than simultaneous immunization.

The new vaccine is now being distributed in considerable amounts to veterinary practitioners in Iowa, Illinois, and several Eastern States, and a better appraisal of its true value can be made when these extended field trials have been completed.

As in the case of anti-hog-cholera serum, the Government has obtained a patent on crystal-violet vaccine with all rights dedicated to the public.

Chapter 2

SWINE ERYSIPELAS

H.W. Schoening, C.G. Grey & O.L. Osteen[1]

[1] *H.W. Schoening is Chief, C.G. Grey is Assistant Veterinarian, and O.L. Osteen is Associate Veterinarian, Pathological Division, Bureau of Animal Industry.*

It was only 20 years ago that swine erysipelas was first definitely recognized in this country. Ten years ago it was found to be an acute herd infection in certain areas. Will it become as serious a disease here as it has been in certain parts of Europe The developments outlined in this article will be watched with interest by producers.

Swine erysipelas has for many years been one of the most important diseases of swine in continental Europe and in England. The causative agent was discovered by Pasteur and Thuillier in 1882 and 1883.[2] Loeffler, working at about the same time, studied the organism but did not publish his observations until 1886.[3] It is of interest to note that in 1879 Koch discovered the mouse septicemia bacillus (*Bacillus murisepticus*),[2] which is considered to be identical with the swine erysipelas bacillus.

---

[2] PREISZ, HUGO. ROTLAUF DER SCHWEINE. *In* Handbuch der pathogenen Mikroorganismen 6: 1-36, illus. 1913.

[3] LOEFFLER. EXPERIMENTELLE UNTERSUCHUNGEN UBER SCHWEINE-ROTHLAUF. [Germany] K. Gsndhtsamt. Arb. 1: [46]-55. 1886.

In the United States, the specific organism of swine erysipelas, technically named *Erysipelothrix rhusiopathiae*, was first isolated in 1921 by Creech,[4] of the Bureau of Animal Industry, from a lesion, or tissue injury, in a hog that came from Texas. The organism was obtained from a specimen of skin showing a typical "diamond skin" lesion. Such lesions, typical of those described in European countries as the result of an infection with swine erysipelas, had been observed in the United States for many years, but the disease was called diamond-skin disease. Swine erysipelas was not considered to be present in this country before the discovery of the organism by Creech. After Creech's discovery other workers isolated the organism from lesions in the joints and some other parts of bodies of swine. It was then recognized definitely that swine erysipelas existed, apparently in a chronic form, in certain parts of the United States.

Beginning in 1930 the disease was recgonised as an acute herd infection in South Dakota, Nebraska, and other States of the Corn Belt, and since that time it has continued to be a more or less serious disease of swine in certain areas in those States.

Nature and Cause of the Disease

Swine erysipelas is an insidious disease, and the manner in which it spreads is not entirely understood. It is quite likely, however, that the disease requires considerable time to make any appreciable headway in certain areas or in a new territory. In certain parts of the United States it has probably existed in a chronic form for many years, gradually increasing in virulence in certain areas until, when favourable conditions prevailed it manifested itself in the explosive, or acute, type.

Breed,[5] reporting on the distribution of swine erysipelas in the United States, stated that the organism had been identified as a cause of swine maladies in 28 of 46 States; from two States no reports were received. While the infection appears to be confined principally

---

[4] CREECH, G.T. THE BACILLUS OF SWINE ERYSIPELAS ISOLATED FROM URTICARIAL LESIONS OF SWINE IN THE UNITED STATES. Amer. Vet. Med. Assoc. Jour. 59: 139-150, illus. 1921.

[5] BREED, FRANK, SWINE ERYSIPELAS, ITS DISTRIBUTION, INCREASING IMPORTANCE AND CONTROL. U.S. Live Stock Sanit. Assoc. Proc. 41: 344-355. 1937.

to the Corn Belt, it perhaps exists in many other States in a chronic, low-grade form.

That the disease flourishes under certain conditions is apparent from the European literature and from observations made in this country. The disease occurs most often during the spring, summer, and fall, but it has been observed in the United States in every month and every season. An explanation for this is that in this country sows farrow every month of the year, and thus there is a continuous supply of new pigs susceptible to the infection.

Swine of all ages are susceptible to the disease, from suckling pigs to adult animals. The causative organism has also been found to affect a variety of birds and animals, including man. Horses, cattle, sheep, dogs, ducks, chickens, turkeys, mud hens, and parrots have been reported to be susceptible. In certain parts of this country, the disease has been of economic importance in sheep and turkeys. That the organism is quite infective to man is evidenced by the number of cases reported in the literature. Veterinarians, butchers, and livestock handlers have frequently been infected. Infection among laboratory workers is not uncommon, while numerous cases have been recorded among workers in bone factories. The so-called fish handlers' disease has been found to be caused by infection with the swine-erysipelas organism, which has been found on the skin of many salt-water fish.

Although it does not bear spores, the erysipelas organism is very resistant to adverse conditions, owing, it is claimed, to a waxy substance it contains. A culture of the organism that was experimentally dried on a glass surface and kept at 98° F. remained alive for a month. In a cool, dark place also it remained active for a month. In smears on glass exposed to direct sunlight, the organism survived only 2 days. Under laboratory conditions in various types of media, it has a very long life. Nocard and Leclainche[6] state that organisms remain alive for 17 days in water. The organism is very sensitive to heat, however. At 111° F. it is destroyed in 4 days, at 125° F. in 15 minutes, and at 130° to 137° F.–far below ordinary cooking temperatures-in several minutes.

---

[6] NOCARD, ED., AND LECLAINCHE, E. LES MALADIES MICROBIENNES DES ANIMAUX. Ed. 3, rev. and enl. 2 v. Paris, 1903.

Living erysipelas organisms have been found in putrid material after 4 months. In the flesh of swine, the organisms are quite resistant to destruction, and Preisz[7] reports living organisms in a carcass that had been buried for 280 days. The organisms are only slowly destroyed by salting and pickling, and they also have been found alive after 26 days in strong brine. Salting hams with salt and saltpeter failed to destroy their virulence in 30 days. Organisms added to pickling fluid were still virulent after 170 days. On the other hand, the organism is not resistant to the action of disinfectants. It is killed by solutions of phenol in 15 minutes, while formalin and ordinary lye readily destroy it.

In areas where the disease is found, the organism exists in the soil as a saprophyte, living on dead or decaying organic matter. Evidence has been presented to show that it can multiply in the soil under certain conditions and that sandy soils rich in lime and humus are especially favourable.

These facts are evidently important in outbreaks of the disease. Since the organism can survive for long periods in certain soils, the recurrence of swine erysipelas can readily be brought about by favourable conditions. It appears that on some farms where infection exists the disease may recur irregularly over a period of several years, though this may not happen on other farms where the soil is similarly infected. No satisfactory explanation has been made for these differences. Once an infection has appeared on a farm, however, a potential danger exists that it will reappear in subsequent years.

It is not definitely known whether infection proceeds directly from animal to animal or whether the organisms excreted by an infected animal must pass some part of their life outside the animal body or otherwise undergo some change before they are capable of reproducing the disease. It is generally agreed that cultures of the organism can reproduce the disease only with the greatest difficulty when injected into swine. It is also generally held that some unknown factor in addition to the organism itself is necessary to bring about infection. The experience of Bureau of Animal Industry pathologists supports this idea. Several years ago, for example, two

---

[7] See reference in footnote 2.

healthy hogs were placed in contact with two hogs affected with a chronic form of swine erysipelas. The four animals were housed in a small enclosure on a concrete floor. After almost 3 months the normal animals remained healthy. Soil was then placed on the concrete floor. About 2½ months later both the normal hogs developed the disease and died within a week of each other. *Erysipelothrix rhusiopathiae* was recovered from the organs of the dead animals.

During an acute attack of the disease, the causative agent can be found in the blood, urine, and feces, and the surroundings of the animals soon become heavily contaminated. Animals affected with the chronic form of the disease may also pass it on to others.

It has been shown that the swine erysipelas organism may be harboured in some parts of the bodies of apparently healthy animals, such as the tonsils and parts of the intestinal tract. Possibly this is a result of a previous infection and recovery, or the organisms may have been picked up from contaminated soil without infection resulting. Such animals may possibly be dangerous to others, or they may subsequently develop the disease themselves.

Symptoms

Acute swine erysipelas is characterized by its sudden onset, and many swine in the herd may be affected at the same time. Only a few may be visibly sick, while a number of others may run high temperatures–105°-110° F. Affected hogs lie in their bedding, but it may be noted that their eyes are clear and active–every move an attendant makes is watched, but they are very reluctant to move themselves. If-forcibly disturbed, they start off with considerable activity but protest with loud squeals. Since the tissues of the joints are involved in the disease process, many of the affected swine are undoubtedly in pain when they walk. They make an effort to keep their feet under them, which makes the backbone appear long and strongly arched. After moving about a bit, they drop down on their bedding again. Where considerable swelling at a joint is noted, there may be exostoses (bony growths), which do not disappear when the disease subsides. Animals thus affected are the so-called knotty-legged hogs, or chronics, which harbour the disease organisms in their joints and may act as spreaders of the infection.

Several of the hogs may die quite suddenly. They may appear well at feeding time one evening and be found dead the next morning.

There have been cases where entire herds have died, but this is rather rare at present in this country although it is not so uncommon in unvaccinated herds in swine erysipelas districts of Europe. As a rule only a few hogs die, some make a complete recovery, and the rest may remain unthrifty chronics.

In hogs acutely in with swine erysipelas, shortness of breath caused by pulmonary edema–a waterlogged condition of the lungs–may be noted. At times swellings about the snout make breathing very difficult. Nausea and vomiting are not uncommon symptoms. Some 24 to 48 hours after the onset of the disease irregular red patches, which are neither tender to the touch nor swollen, may be noted on the lighter parts of the skin. Such areas may remain localized or may enlarge and run together until the greater part of the body surface is involved. Death is sudden, usually preceded by respiratory distress (laboured breathing) brought about by pulmonary edema and heart weakness. The temperature drops, and the mucous membranes become cyanotic (blue).

The so-called diamond skin, skin with regular rhomboidal lesions (Fig. 1), sometimes appears in acute cases in which the affected swine die within 3 days after the onset of the disease. Such lesions on the skin are, however, usually associated with a less severe type of swine erysipelas, in which the symptoms are of a milder character and rapidly subside after the appearance of the characteristic skin eruption. Unless complications set in, hogs affected with the mild type of erysipelas usually recover within 2 weeks. Where the diamond-skin lesions extend over considerable areas, however, there may be a dry gangrenous sloughing of large portions of skin. The ears and tail are often lost in this way. Loss of the tail, which is the more frequent, may be the only apparent evidence of infection, past or present. Skin lesions are difficult to see except on the lighter coloured breeds of hogs or on the light parts of dark breeds.

The swine that do not die of the disease are often left in such a condition that they are unprofitable to the owner. Many have swollen joints, and these animals are discounted by the packer-buyers. Others that do not have enlarged joints may appear dehydrated (dried up), and these are called race-horse pigs by some owners. Such hogs eat a great deal but do not fatten as soon or as well as normal hogs. Joint trouble may appear as an independent manifestation of the disease. All the joints may be enlarged, but those of the knee, hock, and toes are most frequently affected.

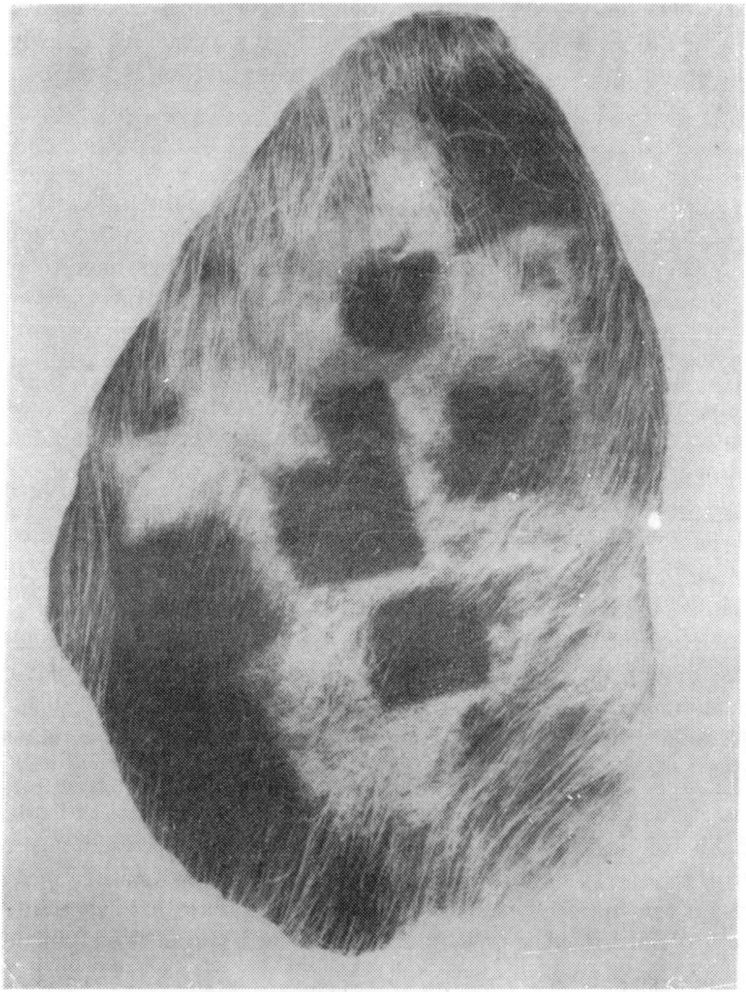

Fig. 1: Rhomboidal, or diamond-shaped, skin lesions of swine erysipelas. This specimen of skin was taken from a hog which was inoculated on October 11 and died on October 14.

At times the only indication of infection in a herd is a dry, scaly eczema (skin eruption), which is nonparasitic in character and fails to clear up in response to changes of feed or the use of dips and oils. Such lesions disappear as a rule upon the administration of specific antiserum, alone or in combination with living culture, as described later.

Diagnosis

The diagnosis of swine erysipelas presents many difficulties, but in areas where it has become prevalent veterinarians, through clinical observations supported by laboratory findings, have been able to recognize it with a fair degree of accuracy. The disease is at times, confusing, however, because it may manifest itself in so many ways. The problem is one for the consideration of a veterinarian.

Symptoms and manifestations that aid in diagnosis are the sudden onset, typical skin discolorations, dehydration (dried-up appearance) of the skin, curled ears, stub tails, evidence of pain on moving, reluctance to move unless forcibly aroused, enlarged joints, scaly eczema, swellings on ears, snout, legs, and elsewhere, sloughed ears and sloughing of patches of skin, and high temperature. The eyes may be clear and the squeal vigorous.

Specimens from suspected outbreaks of swine erysipelas should be forwarded to a diagnostic laboratory for bacteriological examination. Such laboratories are maintained by many of the States to aid in diagnosing and controlling diseases and ailments of livestock and poultry.

Since the definite diagnosis of swine erysipelas is very difficult from a clinical standpoint, attention has been given in recent years to the development of serological methods of diagnosis. These depend on the reaction of whole blood or blood serum in a laboratory test. The Bureau of Animal Industry started working on this problem in 1932 and, after considerable experimentation both in the laboratory and in the field, has developed the rapid-plate agglutination test, which, within limits, has proved a valuable aid in diagnosis.

In using the test it is quite important to recognize its limitations and interpret the results properly. Definitely positive reaction in swine indicates either infection with or exposure to the specific micro-organism. Swine that have recently received infections of the specific antiserum also give positive results as early as 24 hours after the administration of the test, and this reaction may persist for some weeks. The test has little value, therefore, in the case of animals that recently received the specific antiserum.

Positive reactions may possibly be obtained in animals that show no clinical evidence of the disease, which may be explained by the fact that swine erysipelas organisms may be harboured in the body of an animal without producing any visible lesions or symptoms. It is also possible that there may be obscure joint lesions that are the result of erysipelas infection. Experimental work has shown that on a very thorough post mortem examination, most of the apparently normal hogs kept on premises known to be infected and showing a positive reaction to the test will exhibit lesions in one or more joints. By bacteriological examination of a number of these animals it has been possible in most instances to isolate the swine erysipelas organism. Bureau pathologists have found that animals showing visible joint lesions on clinical examination give a strongly positive reaction to the test and that the organisms is easily recovered from such animals. Animals that react less strongly may simply be harbouring it.

Generally speaking, the test is considered to be more applicable to herd diagnosis than to the diagnosis of the disease in individual animals, and for the present its use should be restricted to persons qualified to make proper interpretations. When erysipelas is suspected in a herd, a number of animals should be tested and the diagnosis should not be made until the representative serological picture of the herd can be obtained. The fact should be kept in mind that the chronic form of swine erysipelas may be present in a herd that is also affected with some other acute disease, and a positive reaction does not necessarily shut out the possibility of some other infection also being present.

Control Measures

Since swine erysipelas is propagated in the infected animal and apparently also in the soil, when it appears on a farm to determine the best procedure to follow is a difficult problem. As has been previously stated, the organism may live in the soil for a considerable period, although it can be destroyed in hogpens by the usual cleaning and disinfection.

Since the disease often manifests itself in a low-grade type of infection and since it has been shown that animals affected with this chronic form may under certain circumstances pass it on to normal hogs, it is apparent that such animals should be removed from the herd.

Anti-swine-erysipelas serum has been available for some years, but, while effective, it has certain limitations. The immunity produced by the injection of serum cannot be expected to last more than 2 or 3 weeks. Likewise the serum is effective only when given very early in the acute stage of the disease. After the disease once establishes itself and becomes chronic, the value of the serum is very limited.

In European countries use is made of an active-immunization procedure, which includes administration of both a live culture of the causative agent and hyperimmune serum–the so-called simultaneous method of immunization. This method has not been considered to be applicable for general use in this country because the live culture might set up new centers of infection in cases of mistaken diagnosis of swine erysipelas. In certain sections of the Corn Belt, however, the disease has progressed to such an extent that a large-scale experiment in which the simultaneous method of vaccination is used under restricted conditions is now being conducted cooperatively by several of the State livestock sanitary authorities, the State experiment stations, and the Federal Bureau of Animal Industry. Certain herds are vaccinated with the serum and culture, and accurate records are kept of the results. The plan is to run this project for several years before a final decision is reached as to the applicability of the serum- and-culture method of vaccination in the United States. The results so far have been very satisfactory, but sufficient time has not yet elapsed to get full information.

In handling diseases of swine, owners should always get in contact with State and local veterinarians, and this is particularly important in combating actual or suspected outbreaks of swine erysipelas.

Relation to Arthritis

Considerable experimental work and field observations over a period of years have shown that the swine erysipelas organism has a marked predilection for the joints, even in the early stages of the disease while it is still acute. Arthritis may result from an acute attack of swine erysipelas or from a low-grade infection in which the animal may not be noticeably sick at any time but may later have enlarged joints.

The term "arthritis" designates an inflammation of the joints, whether or not the joint is enlarged. Post mortem examination of a large number of hogs has revealed that those affected with the arthritic form of swine erysipelas may show extensive damage to one or more joints, including the articular surfaces and the joint capsules, with no visible enlargement.

It was demonstrated by Ward[8] as early as 1922 that cases of arthritis in swine were caused by infection with the swine erysipelas organism. Since swine arthritis has become widespread in recent years, it was thought advisable to seek additional information which would give some idea as to the distribution of the disease in various parts of the country. Accordingly, beginning in 1939, specimens of arthritic lesions in swine were obtained from a number of meat-inspection centers in various parts of the country with information as to the origin of the hogs from which the specimens were obtained. Up to the date of writing a total of 572 joints had been received and examined bacteriologically. The swine erysipelas organism was recovered from 444 of these, or 77.62 percent, and it is probable that the percentage would have been higher had it been practical to make extensive cultural tests of all the affected joints. The swine from which these specimens were obtained (swine with erysipelas) had their origin in 114 counties in 16 States (Iowa, Nebraska, Minnesota, South Dakota, Texas, Oklahoma, Arkansas, Tennessee, Mississippi, Alabama, Florida, Virginia, Maryland, Pennsylvania, Kansas, and Missouri) but the greatest number came from the Corn Belt.

Differential Diagnosis

The principal disease with which swine erysipelas might be confused is hog cholera. In acute swine erysipelas the onset of the attack is as a rule more sudden and abrupt and its course more rapid than in hog cholera, and body temperatures are generally higher. In swine erysipelas the animal gives more evidence of pain on being handled than in hog cholera. In swine affected with

---

[8] WARD, ARCHIBALD R. THE ETIOLOGY OF POLYARTHRITIS IN SWINE. Amer. Vet. Med. Assoc. Jour. 61: 155-161. 1922.

erysipelas the eyes remain clear and active, while in those with cholera they become dull and gummy.

There may sometimes be confusion in the picture presented by a post mortem examination, but usually in hog cholera the lymph nodes assume a dark-red or marbled discolouration, while in swine erysipelas there may be little change in colour but marked evidence of edema, though at times a cherry-red to violet discolouration may be noted.

In uncomplicated hog cholera the spleen remains normal in size; in swine erysipelas it usually shows some enlargement. In hog cholera accompanied by certain bacterial infections, however, enlargement of the spleen may be noted.

In hog cholera intestinal lesions are more commonly found in the large intestine. In swine erysipelas they are more commonly observed in the small intestine.

Chapter 3

ENTERITIS OF SWINE

C.N. Dale[1]

[1] *C.N. Dale is Associate Veterinarian, Pathological Division, Bureau of Animal Industry.*

Three very serious forms of intestinal inflammation–necrotic enteritis, swine dysentery, and enteritis of young pigs–are considered here. The first two are especially deadly in combination with hog cholera. Everything that is known about these maladies indicates that the heavy losses they cause could be largely prevented by really good swine husbandry.

The term "enteritis" means an inflammation of the intestines. There are many kinds of enteritis affecting swine, and they vary in intensity. Two of the most serious are necrotic enteritis and swine dysentery.

Necrotic Enteritis

Necrotic enteritis has until recently been considered an infectious disease of swine caused by the micro-organism *Salmonella choleraesuis*. Lately, however, the relation of swine nutrition to the development of this disease has been given prominent attention. The results of investigations now in progress in different sections of the country may clarify the question of the cause of the disease.

Necrotic enteritis has also been called necro, paratyphoid, caseous enteritis, and infectious necrotic enteritis. The term "necrotic enteritis" means an inflammation of the intestines (enteritis) characterized by dead cells or tissue (necrosis). Besides being a specific disease of swine, necrotic enteritis is also a condition associated with other diseases.

The Casual Organism

The disease was first described as early as 1866 (*4*).[2] Later it was associated with hog cholera. After it had been determined that hog cholera was caused by a filtrable virus, further investigation revealed that necrotic enteritis occurred as an independent disease and was caused by the micro-organism *Salmonella choleraesuis* (literally, swine-cholera *Salmonella*) which has also been called *Bacterium choleraesuis, Bacillus suipestifer*, and still later *Salmonella suipestifer*.

In the United States, Murray and associates (*5, 6*) and Biester and associates (*1*) have described extensive investigations of the disease. These investigators were able to produce it in more than 100 pigs by feeding them cultures of the organism. They also isolated the causal organism from all of the field cases that were investigated. A number of other investigators have also shown that necrotic enteritis can be produced by feeding cultures.

Examinations of the bacterial flora of the intestines of apparently healthy swine for the presence of the paratyphoid organism show that relatively few normal pigs harbour the organism. It has been found in a sufficient number, however, to indicate that there may be a carrier type in which the organism is present without causing any appreciable injury. Some change may take place in such an animal that may provide conditions necessary for the organism to become active.

The organism is known to be highly virulent in the presence of hog cholera infection. Thus, when a pig that has been harbouring the *Salmonella* organism without appreciable damage becomes infected with hog cholera virus, the paratyphoid organism invades the body tissues and produces definite lesions. Animals affected with both hog cholera virus and *Salmonella choleraesuis* generally die within 5 to 7 days, whereas hog cholera infection alone usually requires about 15 days to cause death. The combined infections spread from animal to animal, producing a very severe, fatal disease.

---

[2] Italic numbers in parentheses refer to Literature Cited.

S. choleraesuis has been considered to playa part in so-called hog cholera "breaks" and the greatest precautions should be taken in immunizing pigs with hog cholera virus and anti-hog-cholera serum when there is a possibility that this paratyphoid organism is present in the herd.

Knowledge of the role which the *Salmonella choleraesuis* organism plays when associated with hog cholera, although far from complete, is quite extensive, but the information available on its association with other diseases and conditions is more limited. Two forms of the primary *Salmonella choleraesuis* infection are generally recognized–acute, and chronic. It is the chronic form of the infection which has been specifically known as necrotic enteritis.

Symptoms

Necrotic enteritis generally begins with a rise in temperature, diminished appetite, and diarrhoea. A number of factors may bring about variation in the intensity of these symptoms, and during the initial stage the trouble may frequently be diagnosed as hog cholera. If this diagnosis is followed by the administration of hog cholera virus and anti-hog-cholera serum together, the results may be disastrous. Sick pigs and many deaths may be expected. Post mortem examinations will probably reveal lesions, or tissue injuries, due to hog cholera, and the conclusion will be drawn that before the animals were treated the latter disease had progressed too far for the treatment to save them. This is one of the cases in which the services of a veterinarian are needed. Necrotic enteritis in its early stages may be similar to various other acute diseases besides hog cholera, and even with the most careful investigation it may be impossible to determine the exact nature of the trouble. Control measures will be determined by the definiteness and accuracy of the diagnosis.

After the first few days the temperature of pigs affected with necrotic enteritis may return to normal and their appetite improve, but the animals become unthrifty and fail to put on weight normally. Emaciation, weakness, prostration, and death often follow, particularly when no efforts at control are made.

Lesions

It is generally accepted that the lesions revealed by post mortem examination in cases of necrotic enteritis are confined chiefly to the gastrointestinal canal (the stomach and intestines) and are characteristic of the disease. However, many of the lymph glands, particularly those of the stomach and intestines, may be enlarged and reddened and may contain a larger amount of fluid than normal, which gives them a gelatinous appearance. The tonsils may show varying degrees of tissue destruction. The intensity of the involvement of the stomach also varies. In some cases the lining of the stomach is normal; in others the alterations may vary from slight or marked inflammation to extensive destruction of tissue. The small intestines may also fail to reveal any significant injury, but cases are observed in which the lesions vary from slight irritation to definite tissue destruction. The outstanding and most characteristic lesions of the disease are found in the large intestines, the walls of which are generally much thicker than normal. The lining shows the characteristic patches of dead tissue, varying in size from small circular spots to extensive areas involving several feet of the bowel. The entire lining can be easily scraped off. The dead tissue may slough and be mixed with the intestinal contents.

Variation in intensity of the symptoms and lesions is explained by a number of factors.

(1) As in the case of many other disease-producing organisms, different strains of the *Salmonella* organism vary in their virulence or ability to produce disease.

(2) Repeated passage through animals may increase the virulence of the organism.

(3) The severity of the disease may vary with the number of the organisms taken into the animal's body and the frequency with which they are introduced.

(4) Among individual animals and groups of animals there are variations in resistance to infection owing to numerous debilitating factors.

Control Measures

Various remedies have been used for necrotic enteritis, but reports indicate that as a whole they have been unsatisfactory. No known medicinal preparation has sufficient merit to be recommended as a specific treatment.

Experience has shown that it is more profitable to adopt adequate preventive measures than to attempt treatment after the disease has appeared in a herd. Rigid sanitation, as commonly recommended for the control of roundworms in pigs has proved to be quite effective in the prevention of necrotic enteritis. It is advisable to adhere to standard methods of swine production and to supply adequate rations so as to avoid the introduction of factors that might lower resistance to infection. When the disease has become established in a herd, separating the apparently healthy pigs from the sick ones and placing the former in clean quarters or on ground not previously used for swine often checks the spread of the infection.

Relation of Nutrition to Necrotic Enteritis

Much has been written recently on the relation of nutrition to necrotic enteritis in swine. Because of the interpretations given to certain nutritional investigations on rations deficient in pellagra-preventive (P-P) factors, many persons believe that necrotic enteritis is primarily due to a nutritional deficiency and that the addition of liver, yeast, and particularly nicotinic acid to the ration constitutes a cure and preventive. This view overlooks the importance of the *Salmonella choleraesuis* organism and may result in neglect of sanitation as a control measure. The evidence now available does not appear to be sufficient to justify reliance on adequate nutrition alone to control the disease.

On the basis of present knowledge, the situation may be summarized as follows:

1. Necrotic enteritis is a chronic form of *Salmonella choleraesuis* infection.
2. A vitamin deficiency, presumably of nicotinic acid, will produce in swine pellagra or a pellagralike disease, some aspects of which may be like necrotic enteritis.
3. Pigs affected with this vitamin deficiency may be subject to a more severe or extended attack of necrotic enteritis than pigs riot so affected when similarly exposed.
4. When the rations are deficient, nicotinic acid and possibly other factors of the vitamin B complex should be given as a supplement for the prevention and treatment of the deficiency disease.

Swine Dysentery

Although swine dysentery has often been and sometimes still is described as a form of necrotic enteritis. It has become generally recognized as a specific disease. Because of its nature, it has been variously designated as infectious hemorrhagic enteritis, swine typhus, bloody diarrhoea, bloody scours, bloody dysentery, bloody flux, black scours, and colitis (inflammation of the colon).

The disease has been reported in many sections of the country but it appears to be more prevalent in the large swine-producing States of the Midwest than elsewhere. Some idea of its extensiveness may be gained from Hofferd's report (3) that in a single year some veterinarians estimated death losses up to 1,500 head in their respective practices. The history of the majority of outbreaks generally discloses that the affected animals have been either directly or indirectly in contact with sales barns or public stockyards. Enforcement of sanitary regulations at these places has been reported to have been followed by a decrease in the incidence of the disease in swine from these sources.

Symptoms

Swine dysentery is considered to be an acute infectious disease and its outstanding symptom is usually a profuse bloody diarrhoea. The fecal discharge often contains shreds of tissue in addition to varying amounts of blood. The disease starts in a few pigs and more pigs become infected each day. Some go off feed while others show no loss of appetite.

Biester, Schwarte, and McNutt (2) reproduced the disease experimentally in normal pigs by feeding them intestinal tissue and the contents of intestines from affected swine. The pigs showed a rise in temperature from the fourth to the seventh day. Diarrhoea appeared about the sixth day and the elimination of blood a day or two later. On an average, temperatures in swine dysentery do not exceed 105° F. and some do not show an appreciable variation from normal, or 104° F. (In many other acute infectious diseases, such as hog cholera, swine erysipelas, and *Salmonella choleraesuis* infection, the temperature commonly rises to 107° F. or even higher).

Some pigs die suddenly after a couple of days of illness while others linger for 2 weeks or even longer. Pigs that recover are stunted and usually unthrifty. Whiting (7) in 1924 reported that of 192 pigs exposed by feeding or pen contact, 167 developed the disease, while 25 did not show visible symptoms. All the pigs that did not develop the disease were later fed virulent material and remained healthy. Pigs that have recovered are not considered immune and are subject to repeated attacks. In a herd of young pigs 60 percent or more may die. The number of deaths in a herd of older pigs is usually considerably less. Both cholera-immune and cholera-susceptible pigs may be affected. The use of hog cholera virus and anti-hog-cholera serum for immunization of herds in which swine dysentery exists is generally followed by serious losses. Almost total loss of herds affected with swine dysentery has occurred when the disease has been accompanied by hog cholera.

While swine dysentery generally occurs where sanitation is poor and feeding practices questionable, it has been reported in herds kept under good sanitary conditions and fed rations generally recognized as satisfactory.

It has often been observed that the disease frequently occurs in hogs following cattle, including cattle that had been recently brought to the farm. Some observers think that this is merely coincidence, but others have suggested that cattle may be carriers of the disease. Hofferd (3) reports a herd in which the disease recurred whenever corn was added to the diet.

Cause and Lesions

The cause of swine dysentery has not yet been determined. A germ-free filtrate of intestinal tissues from affected pigs has failed to reproduce the disease when fed to healthy swine. A number of different organisms have been isolated from animals affected with the disease which, when fed to normal pigs, also failed to produce the disease.

Laboratory studies have revealed the presence of the organism *Salmonella choleraesuis* in some outbreaks, but in others it has not been found. This organism may not be instrumental in causing the disease, but since it is the cause of necrotic enteritis it seems probable that its presence in cases of swine dysentery may influence the course and final outcome of the dysentery outbreak. Outbreaks in which this organism is not present may respond to control measures differently from those where it is present.

The lesions found on post mortem examination in the early stages are principally in the large intestine. The lining of the cecum and colon is inflamed and bloody. In later stages, shreds and patches of dead tissue are found adhering to the intestinal wall or loose in the fecal contents. The stomach may also show lesions, but the small intestine is not usually involved. When secondary complications set in, lesions in other parts of the body may be found. These vary with the nature of the complicating factors.

Control Measures

Much effort has been given to control of swine dysentery, and many remedial measures have been used. Each has its advocates, and some may be beneficial in lessening the severity of the disease. None has sufficient merit, however, to be recommended as a specific treatment.

A review of the control methods used indicates that preventive measures give the best results. No means of vaccination or immunization is known. Until more is known about the disease it is necessary to rely on sanitation as a means of prevention. Since the exact nature and sources of the causative factor are unknown, sanitary measures must be very broad and must take in all the probable sources of infection. For instance, since cattle or brood sows may be carriers, preventive measures must include them.

Certain procedures may be practical on one farm and others on another. The advice of a veterinarian should be obtained in formulating an adequate and effective scheme of sanitation. Since affected pigs are obviously a common source of infection, extreme caution should be used when swine from the outside are brought to a farm where there is a herd of healthy pigs. The new group should be isolated and quarantined where they may be observed for at least a week, preferably longer, before being added to the healthy group.

If swine dysentary has become established in a herd, the apparently healthy pigs should be separated from the sick ones. When any of the healthy group sicken, they should be removed. On the basis that it is worth while to limit the amount of infected material the pigs can get, some recommend the removal of both groups, sick and healthy, to concrete floors that can be kept thoroughly clean. Others would remove both groups to clean ground. Observations indicate the importance of removing the pigs from the contaminated lots in which they have been running. The contaminated quarters should be cleaned and disinfected before being restocked. It is desirable to wait until the end of the summer before placing pigs in the lots where infection occurred. Good drainage and clean water should be provided. Pigs that have recovered should be sold or for slaughter rather than allowed to remain as a possible source of infection for a new group. At all times attention should be given to standard methods of feeding and proper nutrition.

Sanitary officials have given continuous attention to the formulation and enforcement of regulations to minimize the spread of the disease as a result of the transportation of swine through public stockyards and public sales stables.

When the cause of the disease has been determined, modification of the sanitary measures now employed to control it may be warranted.

Enteritis and Scours in Baby Pigs

The annual loss of young pigs in the United States is very large. On many farms it is not unusual for 50 percent or more of the pigs to die during the first few days of life. Reports indicate that most of these have developed enteritis and scours. The trouble has been attributed almost entirely to faulty nutrition and lack of proper housing, care, and sanitation.

The condition is usually recognized by its common symptom, diarrhoea. The ailment soon spreads to all the pigs in the litter, particularly when the pens are not cleaned and disinfected. The pigs may scour for a few days, stop suckling, and die or become unthrifty.

While it is a common practice to treat the sick pigs by giving some medicinal preparation, such as castor oil or formalin, this procedure offers little chance of success unless primary attention is given to providing clean quarters, proper care and feeding of the mother, and general sanitation.

An enteritis in baby pigs which has some characteristics not common to the so-called scours has been reported. It has been called the little-pig disease or the 3-day-pig disease. The pigs show symptoms of weakness, unsteady gait, emaciation, roughness of hair, and sometimes a wrinkled appearance of the skin, and most of them are droopy and listless. The number of such pigs that have diarrhoea varies.

Post mortem examination reveals a varying degree of enteritis confined largely to the small intestine. The stomach is normal and generally contains curd, which indicates that at birth the pigs were in condition to nurse.

This condition occurs in litters from sows that are fed garbage as well as from sows that are on other rations considered satisfactory. Pigs are usually affected 24 to 72 hours after birth and generally die within 24 to 36 hours after the first symptoms appear. Experimental work so far has failed to reveal the cause. Recent investigations have shown that the blood of affected pigs contains much less blood sugar than that of normal pigs. If the amount of blood sugar was not too low, recoveries often followed injections of glucose solution and forced feeding of milk.

Enteritis Due to Miscellaneous Causes

Inflammation of the intestines is frequently associated with many diseases and ailments caused by protozoa, parasites, bacteria, and viruses, including swine erysipelas, anthrax, and hog cholera. In chronic hog cholera, areas of dead tissue commonly referred to as button ulcers may be observed in the intestines. Various mineral poisons such as lye and copper sulfate also cause enteritis in swine. The control and treatment of these types of enteritis naturally depend on the cause.

Literature Cited

(1) BIESTER, H.E., MURRAY, CHAS., McNUTT, S.H., and PURWIN, PAUL. (1928). STUDIES ON INFECTIOUS ENTERITIS OF SWINE. II. THE PATHOGENESIS OF INFECTIOUS ENTERITIS. Amer. Vet. Med. Assoc. Jour. 72: 1003-1022, illus.

(2) ______SCHWARTE, [L.H.], and McNUTT, [S.H.] (1935). GENERAL CONSIDERATION OF ENTERITIS IN SWINE. Iowa Vet. 6 (5): 5-7, 22-24.

(3) HOFFERD, R.M. (1936). SWINE DYSENTERY IN IOWA FROM A FIELD STANDPOINT. Amer. Vet. Med. Assoc. Jour. 88: 299-310.

(4) HUTYRA, FRANZ, MAREK, JOSEPH, and MANNINGER, RUDOLPH (1938). SPECIAL PATHOLOGY AND THERAPEUTICS OF THE DISEASES OF DOMESTIC ANIMALS. Ed. 4,3 v., illus. London.

(5) MURRAY, CHAS., BIESTER, H.E., PURWIN, PAUL, and McNUTT, S.H. (1927). STUDIES IN INFECTIOUS ENTERITIS OF SWINE. Amer. Vet. Med. Assoc. Jour. 72: 34-65.

(6) MURRAY, CHAS., BIESTER, H.E., PURWIN, PAUL, and McNUTT, S.H. (1929). STUDIES IN INFECTIOUS ENTERITIS OF SWINE. Amer. Vet. Med. Assoc. Jour. 74: 345-356.

(7) WHITING, R.A. (1924). SWINE DYSENTERY. Amer. Vet. Med. Assoc. Jour. 64: 600-610, illus.

Chapter 4
SWINE INFLUENZA

C.N. Dale[1]

[1] *C.N. Dale is Associate Veterinarian, Pathological Division, Bureau of Animal Industry.*

Although swine influenza cannot yet be cured or prevented any more effectively than human influenza can, close study of the disease has led to fundamental discoveries regarding the human malady. The author of this article traces the main points of the story.

Swine influenza is an acute, infectious, and highly contagious disease now known to be caused by the combined action of a filtrable virus and a microscopic organism called *Hemophilus influenzae suis*.

The disease is apparently widespread, but it appears to be more prevalent in the Middle West than elsewhere in the United States. The outbreaks generally occur in the fall and early winter and are more numerous in some years than in others. Observations seem to indicate that improper housing with consequent undue exposure to cold and dampness are predisposing conditions. Such exposure may cause viruses harboured by apparently healthy animals to become active.

Once swine influenza appears, it spreads rapidly through the entire herd, and within 48 to 72 hours after the first pig shows symptoms all the animals may be affected. The pigs become listless and go off feed, and there is marked prostration. The breathing is laboured and jerky, and the animals appear to be very sick and distressed. Coughing is also observed, there may be a watery discharge from the eyes, and the temperature is usually high. After 5 or 6 days of sickness the animals usually recover rapidly. Complications may retard recovery and increase the mortality, which is generally 1 or 2 percent, although losses as high as 10 percent have been reported.

The tissue injuries evident on post mortem examination generally consist of enlarged, watery, and congested lymph glands in the neck and along the bronchial tubes. The lungs show areas of pneumonia which are often confined to the front lobes.

No vaccine is available for use in the field, and there is no known specific medicinal treatment. Affected animals should be provided with clean, well-bedded, comfortable, and properly ventilated quarters. Good care may be helpful in insuring the usual recovery after 6 or 7 days and preventing deaths from secondary complications.

Research on Swine and Human Influenza

The story of the research work that resulted in identifying the cause of swine influenza is exceptionally interesting and indicative of the nature of the disease. Begun in the Bureau of Animal Industry, this research led to a long series of research projects by medical doctors interested in tracking down the cause of human influenza. Eventually the work was amazingly successful. Swine influenza and human influenza were found to be closely related, and today the outlook for combating this major plague of man is better than ever before.

Swine influenza was first described as a specific disease in 1919 by Koen (*11*),[2] a veterinarian in the Bureau of Animal Industry. The description given then may still be used for clinical diagnosis of the disease as it occurs naturally in the field.

Though many disagreed with Koen that such a disease existed, investigations since then have verified his contention, which he expressed in these words:

I have no apologies to offer for my diagnosis of "flu." Last fall and winter we were confronted with a new condition, if not a new

---

[2] Ital numbers in parentheses refer to Literature Cited.

disease. I believe I have as much to support this diagnosis in pigs as the physicians have to support a similar diagnosis in man. The similarity of the epidemic among people and the epizootic among pigs was so close, the reports so frequent, that an outbreak in the family would be followed immediately by an outbreak among the hogs, and vice versa, as to present a most striking coincidence if not suggesting a close relation between the two conditions. It looked like "flu," it presented the identical symptoms of "flu," it terminated like "flu," and until proved it was not "flu" I shall stand by that diagnosis.

During the next 3 or 4 years after Koen's report, the disease as it occurred in the field was described in several publications (*2, 3, 4, 10, 15*). Some of these papers reported bacteriological studies the results of which were negative–that is, the causative agent was not discovered. The descriptions of the disease agreed closely with Koen's, however, although some included symptoms that were not observed by him.

Up to 1931 a few investigations (*8, 14, 30*) had resulted in the isolation of specific micro-organisms that were considered significant as causative agents of the disease, but these findings were not definitely confirmed.

In 1928 McBryde, of the Bureau of Animal Industry, and his associates published a report (*13*) of their investigations on the transmission of the disease. They were able to reproduce the disease by introducing into the noses of healthy pigs mucus from the windpipe and bronchial tubes of animals showing characteristic symptoms of swine influenza. The mucus was mixed with a solution of salt and water. (Such a mixture is called a saline suspension of tracheal and bronchial mucus, and the method of introducing it into the animal is called intranasal instillation). The disease was also transmitted by the same method with nasal instead of tracheal and bronchial secretions from affected pigs. The disease developed in 65 percent of the animals exposed by these means. When healthy pigs were placed in pens with pigs having the disease, 40 percent of the former came down with it.

McBryde and associates also carried out a small number of experiments to determine whether the cause of the disease was a filtrable virus. In all their investigations, however, intranasal instillations of tracheal and bronchial mucus which had been passed through a fine filter to eliminate bacteria failed to produce the disease in healthy swine.

Experiments that Lead to Finding the Cause of Swine Influenza

In 1931 Shope (*17*), of the Rockefeller Institute for Medical Research, reported that swine influenza was caused by the combined action of a filtrable virus and the micro-organism *Hemophilus influenzae* suis.

Shope (*18*) had investigated outbreaks of swine influenza in Iowa in 1928 and again in 1929. Material for laboratory and experimental work was collected from field cases and transported under refrigeration to Princeton, N.J., where the experiments in transmitting the disease to normal swine were conducted. The animals used were obtained in the vicinity of Princeton, an area from which no outbreaks of swine influenza had been reported. Shope called attention to the fact that the normal pigs which McBryde, and his associates had used in their transmission experiments were obtained in a locality where the disease had been prevalent, and suggested that some of these pigs might have had a certain degree of immunity. This may have accounted for the failure of some of them to develop the disease after intranasal instillations of nasal and tracheal material from affected pigs or after being in contact with sick pigs.

By intranasal instillation of small amounts of 10- and 20-percent suspensions of bronchial mucus alone or mixtures of suspensions of bronchial mucus, bronchial lymph glands, and diseased lung, Shope was able to establish swine influenza in normal swine. The disease was produced with eight different strains of the material from Iowa. Shope found that some strains induced a more severe and virulent form of swine influenza than others. The mortality in the experimental cases was higher than that which occurs in natural outbreaks.

Lewis and Shope (*12*) made bacteriological studies of these experimental cases of swine influenza. They also examined, as a control group, animals that were not affected with swine influenza but were either normal or infected with hog cholera or pneumonia. By using a special culture medium for growing bacteria they were able to isolate the same organism from the lung, bronchial exudate, or heart blood of almost all the pigs affected with swine influenza.

They failed to find the organism in any of the normal swine or those infected with hog cholera or pneumonia. They called the organism *Hemophilus infiuenzae suis*.

Efforts were made to test the possibility that *Hemophilus influenzae suis* might cause swine influenza. It was instilled intranasally in several normal pigs. Two became ill and showed symptoms that could be those of swine influenza, but most of the pigs showed no symptoms whatever. The results apparently indicated that the organism alone would not cause swine influenza.

Although the results of the filtration experiments of McBryde and his associates (*13*) pointed very strongly to the conclusion that the cause of the disease was not a filtrable virus, these workers considered that the experiments might have been too few in number to be conclusive. Shope (*19*), therefore, carried on further experiments on the basis of the possibility that the cause of swine influenza was a filtrable virus.

Germ free filtrates of suspensions of lung, bronchial lymph glands, and exudate from pigs affected with swine influenza were instilled intranasally in 10 normal pigs. At the time these experiments were made Shope did not yet know of the role that the *Hemophilus influenzae suis* organism possibly plays in causing swine influenza. Results from 3 of the 10 pigs exposed were interpreted as being negative. The other 7 showed some evidence to indicate that the filtrate had contained an infectious agent. The disease produced was not typical of swine influenza, however, and Shope gave it the name "filtrate disease." It has been produced experimentally many times since, but has never been known to occur naturally. Possibly the disease does occur but because of its mildness goes unrecognized. Usually there is either no rise in temperature or a slight rise that lasts only a day, instead of the high fever lastiag4 to 6 days in typical swine influenza. In the filtrate disease the symptoms of depression, decreased appetite, and altered breathing were slight, and there was no prostration. Occasionally the pigs had a slight cough. Generally the symptoms were so mild as to be noticed only on close observation.

The filtrate disease was very contagious, and symptoms usually appeared in normal swine 2 days after they were placed in contact with pigs already affected. The post mortem lesions of pigs with the disease were generally similar to those in typical cases of swine influenza but not as extensive.

In cases of disease produced the filtrate, bacteriological studies failed to reveal the presence of the *Hemophilus influenzae suis* organism. The difference in this respect between animals affected with the filtrate disease and animals affected with typical swine influenza, suggested that a combination of this organism and a filtrable virus might be necessary to produce typical swine influenza. When mixtures of the filtrate and the *H. influenzae suis* organism were instilled intranasally in normal swine, cases of typical swine influenza developed. The combined action of these two agents was thus established as the cause of the disease.

Immunity Experiments

Shope (*19*) also carried out experiments which indicated that the majority of animals that recover from the experimentally produced disease become immune. He also showed that the serum of the blood of animals that had recovered would neutralize the virus, or make it harmless. In other words, when a definite amount of serum from a pig that has recovered is added to a similar amount of virus, the mixture when instilled intranasally in a normal pig does not produce swine influenza; but when the same amount of serum from a pig that has not had swine influenza is added to the same amount of virus, the mixture when instilled intranasally in a normal pig does produce swine influenza. This so-called neutralization test is used extensively in the studies of influenza as well as of many other filtrable-virus diseases.

In answer to the question whether organisms other than *Hemophilus influenzae suis* act with swine influenza virus to cause the disease, Shope called attention to the relatively large number of cases caused by the virus alone in which none of the organisms that are normally present in the respiratory tract were capable of producing swine influenza.

In citing attempts of investigators to determine the possibility that human influenza also is caused by a filtrable virus, Shope (*19*) suggested that the problem be investigated with the idea that the combined action of the *Hemophilus influenzae* organism commonly found in the human respiratory tract and a filtrable virus might be the cause of influenza in man.

In 1932 Shope (*20*) reported on additional studies on immunity to swine influenza. It was shown that pigs that had recovered from the filtrate disease, acquired either as a result of intranasal instillation of the virus or by contact, became immune to exposure with a mixture of swine influenza virus and the *Hemophilus influenzae suis* organism–that is, they became immune to typical swine influenza. However, the intranasal instillation of the *H. influenzae suis* organism alone did not confer such immunity. Shope also showed that the blood serum of pigs that had recovered from the filtrate disease would neutralize a mixture of virus and *H. influenzae suis.* When such serum was added to the mixture and allowed to stand for an hour, the combined materials failed to produce swine influenza when instilled intranasally into susceptible pigs, but if serum from normal pigs was used the combined material would produce the disease.

It was also demonstrated that when swine influenza virus alone was injected into the muscles of pigs, instead of being introduced by the other methods described, it would not produce swine influenza even though the *Hemophilus influenzae suis* organism was present in the respiratory passages. Although pigs thus treated were not affected with the disease, they became immune.

Cause of Human Influenza Determined

In 1933 Smith, of the National Institute for Medical Research, London, and his associates (*29*) reported the production of a disease in ferrets by the intranasal instillation of bacteria-free filtrates of throat washings obtained from human patients with influenza. The disease was also transmitted from sick to healthy ferrets either by contact or by direct transfer of nasal washings. Ferrets that had recovered from the disease were found to be immune for some time to subsequent infection with the same strain of virus. As Shope had shown that serum from swine that had recovered from swine influenza would neutralize swine influenza virus, these investigators showed that the serum from ferrets that had recovered from human influenza would likewise neutralize the human influenza virus, as evidenced by the failure of the disease to develop in ferrets when a mixture of the virus and serum were instilled intranasally. By similar tests these workers also demonstrated that serum from human patients after their recovery from influenza would neutralize the human influenza virus, although the results of these tests were not always constant. It was suggested that this inconstancy was a result of their inability to measure the amount of virus in the infective material and the number of neutralizing bodies in the serum used in the mixtures.

Comparative Studies of Swine and Human Viruses

Smith obtained, for comparative studies, samples of the swine influenza virus and the *Hemophilus influenzae suis* organisms with which Shope had produced influenza in swine. When the swine influenza virus was instilled intranasally in ferrets, it produced a disease that was indistinguishable in its symptoms from that produced by the human influenza virus. The nature of the disease in ferrets was not altered when the swine influenza organism was injected together with the swine influenza virus. When cross-immunity tests in ferrets were made, it was found that the animals that had recovered from the disease produced by the swine virus were solidly immune to the human strain of virus but that ferrets that had recovered from the disease produced by the human virus were not completely immune to the swine virus. The tests did, however, indicate a close relationship between the two strains of viruses.

In 1934 Shope (*21*) showed that the swine influenza virus produces a more severe type of disease in ferrets if it is instilled intranasally when the animals are under ether anesthesia. A specific type of pneumonia would develop in ferrets thus exposed.

Later in 1934, Andrewes, of the National Institute for Medical Research, London, and his associates (*1*) were able to produce a specific disease in mice with both the human and the swine viruses by injecting them intranasally into these animals when they were under ether anesthesia. As in ferrets, the disease produced in mice by the mixture of swine influenza virus and the *Hemophilus influenzae suis* organism, which is necessary for producing typical swine influenza in swine, was no different from that produced by the swine influenza virus alone. It was also shown that mice could be used to test sera for the presence of bodies that would neutralize the viruses. This neutralization test in mice has been used extensively in the studies of influenza that have been carried on since that time.

During the next few years, strains of human influenza virus other than the one isolated by Smith were recovered from outbreaks of influenza in other countries. At first it was thought that these strains were identical, but in 1938 neutralization and immunity tests with 28 strains showed that they were not all alike, although they were definitely related (*28*).

In 1935 Shope (22) reported that swine influenza virus could be established directly in mice by intranasal instillation of suspensions of affected swine lung. At the same time experiments showed that mice immunized against specific strains of the human virus were resistant to swine influenza virus. Similar tests showed that mice immunized against the swine influenza virus were resistant to a specific strain of the human virus. Mouse neutralization tests made later showed that various strains of human virus acted differently in their ability to produce antibodies against swine influenza virus.

After the development of the neutralization test in mice, by which the quantity of protective antibodies in human and animal sera could be measured, and the perfecting of the method of isolating the viruses in laboratory animals which proved that there were different strains, it was not long before a vast amount of information resulting from such tests became available for study. Even though a large part of the work has pertained to human influenza, it has often been necessary to include somewhat parallel investigations with the swine influenza virus. Some of the work on human influenza seems particularly significant in the study of swine influenza and indicates the necessity for further research to extend the knowledge of the relationship between the two viruses.

Results of experiments were reported which showed that the sera of animals exposed several times, instead of only once, to either the human or the swine virus contained antibodies against both viruses (*7*).

The results of mouse neutralization tests with samples of human sera showed that a large majority of the samples contained neutralizing bodies (antibodies) against a specific human strain of virus (*6*). A very high proportion of the samples from adults neutralized swine influenza virus, but the samples from children under 12 years of age seldom did (*23*). Two explanations have been offered for the presence of larger amounts of swine influenza antibodies in the sera of adults than of children. One is that the adults have been exposed to human influenza several times, and as a result, as has been shown in experimental animals, antibodies against swine influenza virus have been produced, whereas in children, who presumably have been subjected to only a single attack, such antibodies have not been produced. The other explanation is that the swine influenza virus is the surviving type of the agent that was primarily responsible for the outbreak of human influenza in 1918. Adults who had been exposed to or infected with the virus as it existed at that time developed antibodies against it. Such antibodies were not present in the sera of children, who had not been exposed to that virus.

Neutralization tests with sera from persons living on the island of St. Helena, where an outbreak of influenza occurred in 1936 (*31*), support the idea that the amount of swine influenza antibodies in human serum may increase following an attack of influenza caused by a supposedly human type of virus. No outbreak of influenza had occurred on this island from 1917 to 1921. The sera of individuals living on the island during that period had slight or negligible antibodies when tested in 1935 for either a specific strain of human virus or swine influenza virus. Several months after the 1936 outbreak, tests of the sera from the same individuals revealed that not only had the antibodies for the human virus increased but also that antibodies for the swine strain had been acquired by persons who had none when tested in 1935.

While serological investigations may have no immediately practical application–at least so far–to the handling of field outbreaks of influenza in swine, they serve as basic information for veterinarians and others who are concerned with the origin, spread, and distribution of the swine disease.

Action of the Human Influenza Virus in Swine

The human influenza virus when instilled intranasally in young pigs produced a mild illness, and a mixture of the virus and swine influenza organisms produced a more severe illness (*27*). Further investigations (*27*) of the ability of the human influenza virus to produce disease in swine showed that while the symptoms and lesions in swine infected with the human virus alone were indistinguishable from those produced by the swine virus alone, some differences were observed between typical swine influenza and the disease produced by a mixture of the human virus and *Hemophilus influenzae suis*. As outbreaks of a disease with which the human influenza virus is associated may occur in swine in the field, these differences should be recognized, for otherwise such outbreaks may not be correctly diagnosed or may be considered to be a typical cases of swine influenza. In experimental cases produced by the mixture of the human virus and *H. influenzae suis*, the period of fever may be 2 or 3 days shorter than in swine influenza. The animals are depressed and their appetites diminished, but while they may appear listless they do not show the marked prostration so often seen in swine influenza. Respiratory symptoms occur but are less marked than in swine influenza. The results of a few experiments suggest that infection in swine with the human virus may not be readily transmitted to normal swine by contact, but this may not be true in outbreaks in the field.

The actual isolation of the human virus from swine in field outbreaks has not yet been reported. However, mouse neutralization tests of sera from field herds of swine indicate that they are attacked by the human virus (*24*). Sera from older pigs that were on farms during a period when people living there had been affected with the human influenza virus contained antibodies that neutralized the human virus but not the swine virus. Younger swine, farrowed long after the cases of human influenza, did not contain antibodies for either the human or the swine virus.

Other Recent Findings

Scott (*16*), of the School of Veterinary Medicine of the University of Pennsylvania, found that relatively large doses of the hemorrhagic septicemia organism when instilled intranasally produced no illness in normal swine, whereas a mixture of a small amount of the organism and swine influenza virus produced clinical symptoms that resembled swine influenza. Only a slight feverish reaction resulted from the intranasal instillation of the swine influenza virus alone.

It is known that in the field hemorrhagic septicemia infection is often secondary to or associated with hog cholera. Little is known about the frequency of herd outbreaks in which hemorrhagic septicemia infection may be secondary to or associated with swine influenza.

It has been reported that lungworm larvae may act as a reservoir of swine influenza virus from one season to the next (*25*). The virus is harboured by lungworm larvae from pigs with swine influenza during their development in their intermediate host, the earthworm. After the parasite reaches the respiratory tract of a new swine host, swine influenza occurs when the virus is liberated or made active by certain stimuli.

More recently it has been reported that such stimuli to be effective must occur during the late fall, winter, or early spring months (*26*). During the summer these stimuli have not caused swine influenza in pigs harbouring lungworms that are carriers of swine influenza virus. As yet there is no explanation for this seasonal variation, but some of the endocrine glands are suspected of being responsible.

Suggested Nomenclature

In order that there may be a common terminology to apply to various types of influenza, it has been suggested (*9*) that the type of virus isolated by Smith be called influenza virus A and the disease it causes influenza A. It was also suggested that since the group of diseases commonly called influenza are not all caused by influenza virus A, the names influenza Virus B, C, etc., be given to each specific virus isolated as the cause of the disease it produces. The virus isolated by Francis (*5*), of the New York University College of Medicine, is thus called influenza virus B and produces the disease influenza B. This terminology applies only to human influenza and not to influenza in animals. Consequently the term "swine influenza virus" is retained.

Literature Cited

(1) ANDREWES, C.H., LAIDLAW, P.P., and SMITH, WILSON (1934). THE SUSCEPTIBILITY OF MICE TO THE VIRUSES OF HUMAN AND SWINE INFLUENZA. Lancet [London] 227: 859-862.

(2) DIMOCK, W.W., and HEALY, D.J. (1922). INFLUENZA OF SWINE, "HOG FLU," BRONCHO-PNEUMONIA. North Amer. Vet. 3: 138-141.

(3) DORSET, M., McBRYDE, C.N., and NILES, W.B. (1922). REMARKS ON "HOG FLU." Amer. Vet. Med. Assoc. Jour. 62: 162—171.

(4) DREHER, W.H. (1922). SWINE DISEASES AS WE FIND THEM IN THE FIELD. Amer. Vet. Med. Assoc. Jour. 61: 178-181.

(5) FRANCIS, THOMAS, Jr. (1940). A NEW TYPE OF VIRUS FROM EPIDEMIC INFLUENZA. Science 92: 405- 408.

(6) FRANCIS, THOMAS, Jr., and MAGILL, T.P. (1936). THE INCIDENCE OF NEUTRALIZING ANTIBODIES FOR HUMAN INFLUENZA VIRUS IN THE SERUM OF HUMAN INDIVIDUALS OF DIFFERENT AGES. Jour. Expt. Med. 63: 655-668, illus.

(7) _____and SHOPE, RICHARD E. (1936). NEUTRALIZATION TESTS WITH SERA OF CONVALESCENT OR IMMUNIZED ANIMALS AND

THE VIRUSES OF SWINE AND HUMAN INFLUENZA. Jour. Expt. Med. 63: 645-653.

(8) FULTON, J.S. (1930). HOG INFLUENZA. Amer. Vet. Med. Assoc. Jour. 77: 368-371.

(9) HORSFALL, F.L., Jr., LENNETTE, E.H., RICKARD, E.R., and Others (1940). THE NOMENCLATURE OF INFLUENZA. Lancet [London] 239: 413-414.

(10) KINSLEY, A.T. (1923). SWINE "FLU." Vet. Med. 18: 314.

(11) KOEN, I.S. (1919). A PRACTICAL METHOD FOR FIELD DIAGNOSIS OF SWINE DISEASES. Amer. Jour. Vet. Med. 14: 468-470.

(12) LEWIS, PAUL A., and SHOPE, RICHARD E. (1931). SWINE INFLUENZA. II. A HEMOPHILIC BACILLUS FROM THE RESPIRATORY TRACT OF INFECTED SWINE. Jour. Expt. Med. 54: 361-371.

(13) McBRYDE, C.N., NILES, W.B., and MOSKEY, H.E. (1928). INVESTIGATIONS ON THE TRANSMISSION AND ETIOLOGY OF HOG FLU. Amer. Vet. Med. Assoc. Jour. 73: 331-346.

(14) MURRAY, CHARLES (1920). NOTES ON A MICROCOCCUS ISOLATED FROM CASES OF BRONCHO-PNEUMONIA (so-CALLED "FLU") OF SWINE. Amer. Vet. Med. Assoc. Jour., 57: 539-542.

(15) _____(1921). WHAT IS HOG "FLU." Wallace's Farmer 46: [371], illus.

(16) SCOTT, JOSEPH P. (1938). SWINE INFLUENZA. 13th Internatl. Vet. Cong. Proc. 1: 479-487.

(17) SHOPE, RICHARD E. (1931). THE ETIOLOGY OF SWINE INFLUENZA. Science 73: 214-215.

(18) _____(1931). SWINE INFLUENZA. I. EXPERIMENTAL TRANSMISSION AND PATHOLOGY. Jour. Expt. Med. 54: 349-358.

(19) _____(1931). SWINE INFLUENZA. III. FILTRATION EXPERIMENTS AND ETIOLOGY. Jour. Expt. Med. 54: 373-385.

(20) _____(1932). STUDIES ON IMMUNITY TO SWINE INFLUENZA. Jour. Expt. Med. 56: 575-585.

(21) _____(1934). THE INFECTION OF FERRETS WITH SWINE INFLUENZA VIRUS. Jour. Expt. Med. 60: 49-61.

(22) _____(1935). THE INFECTION OF MICE WITH SWINE INFLUENZA VIRUS. Jour. Expt. Med. 62: 561-572.

(23) _____(1936). THE INCIDENCE OF NEUTRALIZING ANTIBODIES FOR SWINE INFLUENZA. VIRUS IN THE SERA OF HUMAN BEINGS OF DIFFERENT AGES. Jour. Expt. Med. 63: 669-684, illus.

(24) _____(1938). SEROLOGICAL EVIDENCE FOR THE OCCURRENCE OF INFECTION WITH HUMAN INFLUENZA VIRUS IN SWINE. Jour. Expt. Med. 67: 739-748.

(25) _____(1939). AN INTERMEDIATE HOST FOR THE SWINE INFLUENZA VIRUS. Science 89: 441-442.

(26) _____(1941). THE INFLUENCE OF HOST AND INTERMEDIATE RESERVOIR HOST IN DETERMINING THE EPIDEMIOLOGIC PATTERN OF BOVINE PSEUDORABIES AND SWINE INFLUENZA. *In* Problems, and Trends in Virus Research, Univ. Pa. Bicentennial Conf., pp. 55-66.

(27) SHOPE, RICHARD E., and FRANCIS THOMAS, Jr. (1936). THE SUSCEPTIBILITY OF SWINE TO THE VIRUS OF HUMAN INFLUENZA. Jour. Expt. Med. 64: 791-801, illus.

(28) SMITH, WILSON, and ANDREWES, C.H. (1938). SEROLOGICAL RACES OF INFLUENZA VIRUS. Brit. Jour. Expt. Path. 19: 293-314, illus.

(29)_____ANDREWES, C.H., and LAIDLAW, P.P. (1933). A VIRUS OBTAINED FROM INFLUENZA. PATIENTS. Lancet [London] 225: 66-68, illus.

(30) SPRAY, ROBB SPAULDING (1922). THE BACTERIA IN NORMAL AND DISEASED LUNGS OF SWINE. Jour. Infec. Dis. 31: 10-21.

(31) STUART-HARRIS, C.H., ANDREWES, C.H., SMITH, WILSON, and others (1938). A STUDY OF EPIDEMIC INFLUENZA, WITH SPECIAL REFERENCE TO THE 1936-7 EPIDEMIC. [Gt. Brit.] Med. Res. Council, Spec. Rpt. Ser. 228, 151 pp., illus.

Chapter 5

MISCELLANEOUS DISEASES OF SWINE

G.T. Creech[1]

[1] *G.T. Creech is Senior Veterinarian, Pathological Division, Bureau of Animal Industry.*

Facts regarding the symptoms, causes, prevention, and (where possible) treatment of swine pox, infectious arthritis, necrotic rhinitis and stomatitis, posterior paralysis, pneumonia, mastitis, various skin inflammations, and swine plague are given in this article.

Swine Pox

Available information indicates that swine pox has probably existed in European countries for a century or more, but the disease has been definitely recognized in this country for only a little over a decade. McNutt, Murray, and Purwin[2] were among the first to recognize and describe the disease in the United States (1928). Since that time others have investigated it, and recently Shope[3] made rather

[2] McNUTT, S.H., MURRAY, CHAS., and PURWIN, PAUL. SWINE POX. Amer. Vet. Med. Assoc. Jour. 74: 752-761, illus. 1929.

[3] SHOPE, RICHARD E. SWINE POX. Arch. f. die Gesam. Virusforsch. 1: 457-467, illus. 1940; [Reprinted in Rockefeller Inst. Med. Res. Studies 116: 397-408].

detailed studies with particular reference to the nature of the virus, or causative agent. The disease is fairly prevalent in the Middle West and has also been encountered to some extent in the Eastern States.

Swine pox is an infectious disease which is now known to be caused by two types of virus. This is evidenced by the fact that swine that have recovered from the disease are immune to the particular type of virus that caused the attack but are still susceptible to the other type of virus, to which they have not been exposed. The disease is observed most frequently in very young animals, particularly sucking pigs, and seldom is seen in pigs more than 6 months of age. Some pigs are more resistant to the infection than others; when the pigs in a herd are affected, as a rule there win be a few that show no evidence of the disease.

The symptoms manifested in swine pox depend on the severity of the attack. In the more acute form there are well-developed symptoms and skin lesions, but in the milder form only slight manifestations of the disease may appear. The symptoms commonly observed in the more acute form are dullness, weakness, loss of appetite, chills, and a rise of several degrees in temperature. In many cases there is a catarrhal discharge from the eyes and nose. In some of the milder cases the skin lesions may develop to some extent without evidence of any general disturbance of the system.

The skin lesions are first noticeable as small reddish areas on various parts of the body, most frequently on the face and ears, in the armpits, on the inner surface of the thighs, and on the abdomen. In the more severe cases, much of the skin of the body may be involved, including that of the neck, shoulders, sides, and back. The size of the reddened areas may increase to that of a dime or become even larger. They become raised above the surface of the surrounding skin, developing into rather definite nodular areas, or papules (pimples). After several days, small vesicles, or blisters, are seen at the centers of the papules. The vesicles at first contain a clear fluid which later becomes cloudy and puslike. The blisters cause itching and in rubbing them the pig ruptures many of the vesicles, which may bleed and some of which may become more or less fused together. After several more days, the pustules tend to dry up and the centers shrink and become depressed or craterlike (Fig. 1). Later dark scabs form and these eventually drop off or are rubbed off by the pig.

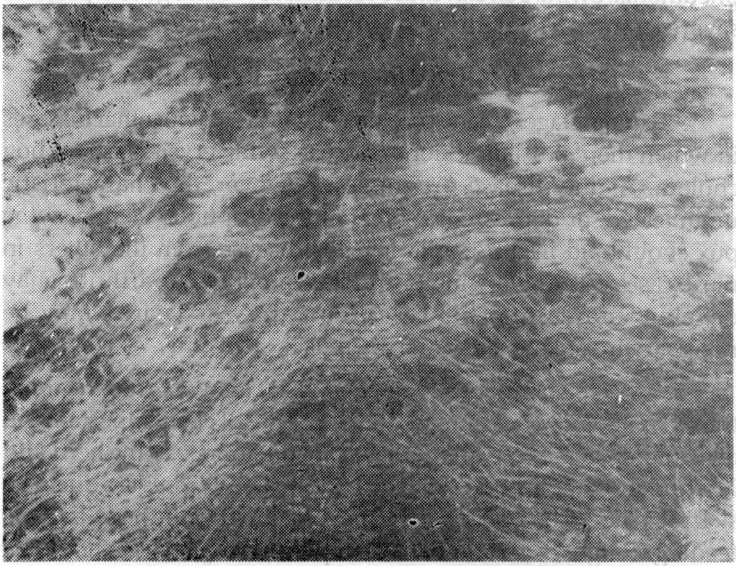

Fig. 1: Skin lesions in a typical case of swine pox. Note the characteristic crater-like centers of the eruptions. (Courtesy of H.E. Biester, Iowa Agricultural Experiment Station).

In some of the more acute cases, vesicles which subsequently become ulcers and destroy tissue may form in the mucous lining of the mouth, pharynx (in the upper part of the throat), stomach, intestinal tract, and possibly the trachea (windpipe) and bronchial tubes as well. Certain of the lymph glands, such as the inguinal, in the groin, may become enlarged.

Microscopically, the skin lesions or injuries in swine pox are seen to be of an acute inflammatory nature, involving both the inner and outer layers (dermis and epidermis), in which there are heavy infiltrations of serum and inflammatory cells (white cells) from the blood stream. As a result of the infiltration of serum and cells, the skin in the areas involved is swollen and thickened.

The symptoms, including the skin lesions, and the general course of the disease may vary considerably in individual pigs, the final outcome in many cases depending on possible complications, such as severe diarrhoea with rapid exhaustion, bronchitis, and pneumonia. Swine pox can cause considerable damage and possibly severe losses, particularly among the suckling pigs of a herd.

Diagnosis, Treatment, and Prevention

At certain stages, swine pox may be confused with other diseases in which there are skin lesions, such as swine erysipelas and hog cholera. As the disease progresses, however, the characteristic umbilicated, or depressed, centers of the eruptions seen in swine pox should aid in differentiating this disease from the others in most cases. Also, in swine erysipelas lameness or arthritis may develop. In questionable cases laboratory assistance may be necessary in making a definite diagnosis.

No specific treatment for swine pox is known. Proper care of the sick pigs and strict sanitary measures are of chief importance in controlling the disease after it has gained entrance to the herd and in avoiding complications, to which the heaviest losses are due. The sick pigs should be isolated from the remainder of the herd, and the feeding troughs, floors, and walls of pens or hog houses should be thoroughly cleaned and disinfected. Hot lye solution is a very satisfactory disinfectant. The healthy pigs should be removed to clean, sanitary quarters, which in the winter season should be warm and have plenty of bedding. All pigs should have good nourishing food and access to a plentiful supply of fresh drinking water. Proper attention to the herd during the period of sickness will reduce losses from swine pox very considerably.

Shope and other investigators made the important observation that swine pox is not transmitted from sick to healthy pigs by contact. They found that lice carry the virus from animal to animal and may spread the disease throughout an entire herd. The most important preventive measure consists in the prompt and effective eradication of hog lice.

Infectious Arthritis

Infectious arthritis, commonly referred to as joint ill or navel ill, is an acute infectious disease of recently farrowed pigs that has been known to hog raisers for a long time. As a rule the disease occurs sporadically and may cause heavy losses in some herds. The disease is characterized by inflammatory changes, with possible abscess formation of the umbilical, or navel, tissues and inflammation of the joints.

Infectious arthritis is caused by different types of germ infections. A number of pyogenic, or pus-producing, micro-organisms, including streptococci, staphylococci, and certain types of the colon bacillus, have been found associated with the disease. In most cases the infecting organisms gain entrance to the body through the tender navel cord soon after birth. They are distributed through the tissues by the blood stream and eventually reach the joints, where they tend to become localized.

While navel ill in young pigs is due specifically to certain types of infection, there are also a number of contributing or predisposing causes, such as improper care, damp, insanitary quarters, and lack of proper bedding on concrete floors.

The manifestations of the disease depend somewhat on the virulence and extent of the infection in individual pigs. In the more typical cases some evidence of inflammation of the umbilicus, or navel, is frequently observed, and in some there are accumulations of pus. The joints are definitely swollen, and when they are opened, the synovial, or joint, membranes will be found to be distended, with a turbid or coagulated fluid. In the late stages the joint tissues may be infiltrated with pus. Occasionally the infection will be carried by the circulation to such organs as the liver and spleen, where abscesses may form.

The symptoms of the disease appear most frequently a few days after birth or during the first week of life, but they may be observed occasionally during the second or third week. At first a disinclination to suckle, dullness, and possibly constipation may be noted in the affected pigs, and these symptoms may be followed by diarrhoea. There is evidence of lameness, and on examination one or more of the joints will be found to be swollen, hot, and painful. Usually there is marked weakness and rapid emaciation, and as a rule the course of the disease is rather brief, death occurring about the second or third day.

In diagnosing infectious arthritis it may be necessary to differentiate the disease from certain others in which joint lesions, with resulting lameness, may also occur, such as swine erysipelas or swine brucellosis. The presence of associated navel lesions should aid in reaching a definite diagnosis.

No specific treatment for the condition after the pigs have become infected is known. Preventive measures are, therefore, of greatest importance. Infection in most cases follows soiling of the stump of the sensitive navel cord with contaminated material from bedding or floors, a fact that should be emphasized. Consequently, the first and most important step in the prevention of infection of young pigs is to provide clean quarters for sows at farrowing time. In fact infectious arthritis can probably be largely prevented in most herds by providing sanitary surroundings at farrowing time. Clean bedding should be provided for the sow and litter and should be changed rather frequently. The young pigs should be prevented from lying directly on concrete floors. As a definite and practical preventive measure, the navel cords of all pigs should be tied with sterile cord, the end of the cord clipped, and the stump dipped in tincture of iodine as soon as practicable after birth.

During the first few days after farrowing, or until the navel cord has dried up and fallen off it would also be well to examine the pigs from time to time in order to detect any possible indications of infection as evidenced by inflammation of the navel. When inflammation is noted, the navel should be washed in warm water to which a small amount of cresol has been added and then dusted with powdered alum. Pigs showing evidence of sickness should be given a physic of either Epsom salt or raw linseed oil and should be housed in a warm, dry place, particularly in cold weather. Occasionally pigs seem to recovery from the infection, particularly when turned out to pasture, but in a number of such cases a recurrence of the arthritis when the pigs were again housed for fattening has been noted.

In handling the herd as a whole, it is always a good sanitary procedure on removing hogs from the various pens and hog houses to cleanse and disinfect such quarters thoroughly before they are occupied again. A 4-percent hot lye solution may be used as a disinfectant for cleaning and scrubbing the woodwork, floors, etc. Several hours after they are cleaned with the lye, thoroughly wash the quarters with clean water.

Necrotic Rhinitis and Stomatitis

Necrotic rhinitis, or so-called bull nose, is most frequently observed in growing pigs. It is characterized by swelling and enlargement of the tissues of the nose and face, including the bony structures, which results in more or less deformity. There are also necrosis, or destruction, and sloughing of the tissues of the snout, lips, and other parts of the mouth.

The condition is infectious and is caused by a micro-organism, *Actinomyces necrophorus.*

Rather widespread in nature, the organisms gain entrance to the tissues in the region of the nose or mouth through wounds or abrasions that may result from blows or fighting, or they enter the lips and gums through injuries caused by certain types of rough feed or by foreign objects such as wire. Filthy surroundings or generally insanitary conditions are very conducive to bull nose infection.

One of the first symptoms noted is a partial loss of appetite. The affected pigs may root in their feed but eat very little. Because the pigs sneeze repeatedly, the condition is commonly referred to by hog owners as sniffles. In sneezing, a certain amount of bloody discharge mixed with clumps of dead tissue may be expelled from the nasal cavities. Many of the affected pigs make a peculiar blowing sound that is considered one of the characteristics of the disease. The snout is enlarged, and lumps or swellings may be seen on some parts of the face. When some of these swellings are opened they are found to contain a cheeselike material which has a disagreeable odour. In many cases the bones of the nose and face are destroyed. In the late stages of the infection the pigs eat with difficulty and gradually become weak and emaciated. If the infection is permitted to continue, it will eventually result in the death of the animals.

Treatment may be undertaken in the very early stages while the swellings on the face are still small or before the infection becomes deep-seated. The swellings should be opened, and as much as possible of the puslike material should be removed. Half-strength tincture of iodine should then be injected into the cavity. It should be understood, however, that after the infection is fairly well established, treatment is in most cases very unsatisfactory or of little avail, largely on account of the involvement and destruction of the bones of the nose and face. In such cases the affected pigs should be destroyed.

If the affected pigs are not destroyed, they should be placed in separate quarters. Occasionally a pig may recover, but as a rule it is advisable to destroy all pigs showing well-marked evidence of infection. The noninfected pigs should be removed to clean sanitary surroundings to prevent the further spread of the infection. The quarters previously occupied by the pigs should be thoroughly cleaned and disinfected, with particular attention to mudholes or damp insanitary parts of hog lots. The use of open pens or hog lots that have been left unoccupied and exposed to direct sunlight for a considerable period and will also prove helpful in overcoming such infections.

Necrotic stomatitis, a type of sore mouth in suckling pigs, is thought to be due to the same cause as necrotic rhinitis. The affected pigs are observed to suckle with some difficulty, and on examining the mouth ulcerated areas with reddish borders and yellowish-white centers are noticeable on the gums, lips, and palate. There are necrosis and sloughing of the tissues, with which a disagreeable odour is associated. Owing to the difficulty of eating as a result of soreness and pain, the affected pigs soon become weak and emaciated.

Treatment of infectious sore mouth, as of necrotic rhinitis, is usually unsatisfactory after the infection has become well established, and in both these conditions primary attention should be directed toward prevention by proper sanitation.

Goiter (Hariless Pigs)

Goiter in swine is rather widely distributed in some parts of the United States, particularly in the Northwest and the Great Lakes region. For a long time the cause of goiter remained obscure, but the disease is now definitely known to be caused by deficiency of iodine in the ration of the sow during the period of pregnancy.

Paralysis of Hindquaters

Paralysis of the hindquarters is a rather common manifestation of disease in swine. In many cases the cause is obscure, though there have been a number of theories concerning it, and treatment is unsatisfactory.

It has been fairly definitely determined that vitamin deficiencies, including that of vitamin A and possibly others, may cause paralysis in swine. It has also been found that certain inflammatory conditions of the spinal cord and related nerve tissues, presumably due to some type of germ infection, may cause posterior paralysis. In growing pigs and pregnant brood sows, an inadequate mineral supply may result in a soft condition of the bones, making them subject to fracture, and such fractures, either of the spinal vertebrae or of the femur, or thigh bone, may cause symptoms that very closely resemble posterior paralysis. Paralysis sometimes follows parturition in sows that are in run-down condition and are being suckled heavily. Diseased conditions of the spinal cord or vertebrae, such as those caused by tumors, abscesses, and tuberculosis, may result in paralysis. It is also claimed that parasites, such as the kidney worm of swine, may occasionally invade the loin muscles and cause posterior paralysis. Other conditions, such as lack of exercise, lumbago, and rheumatism, are said to be contributing causes.

As a rule posterior paralysis develops gradually. The first indications are a wobbly or unsteady gait and inability of the animal to control the hindquarters. As the condition progresses, walking becomes more difficult and weakness of the hindquarters more pronounced. Finally the animal is unable to stand on the hind feet and drags the hindquarters when forced to move (Fig. 2). In exceptional cases, the first symptoms noted may be stamping of the hind feet, or a quick raising or lowering of the feet, which may be followed shortly by definite evidence of paralytic changes and loss of control of the hindquarters. For a time the affected animal may have a very good appetite and fail to show any other functional disturbance. If the paralysis cannot be remedied, however, the animal will eventually refuse feed, develop constipation, and show a general loss of condition.

Because the cause in many cases is obscure, treatment of posterior paralysis is not very satisfactory. Regardless of the cause, however, the first step in treatment is to make the animal as comfortable as possible. If there is evidence of constipation, a dose of Epsom salts or linseed oil should be given. Feed a light diet, such as slop made of milk and bran, and provide clean bedding and an ample supply of fresh drinking water. In some cases massaging of the loin muscles with a good liniment may prove beneficial. If the affected animals is a sow sucking a large litter, the pigs should be weaned. A ration consisting of crushed wheat, bran, and milk made into a slop will prove beneficial in restoring the animal's vitality, depleted by heavy suckling. Sows that have recently farrowed should also have plenty of green feed in the ration to provide the necessary vitamins.

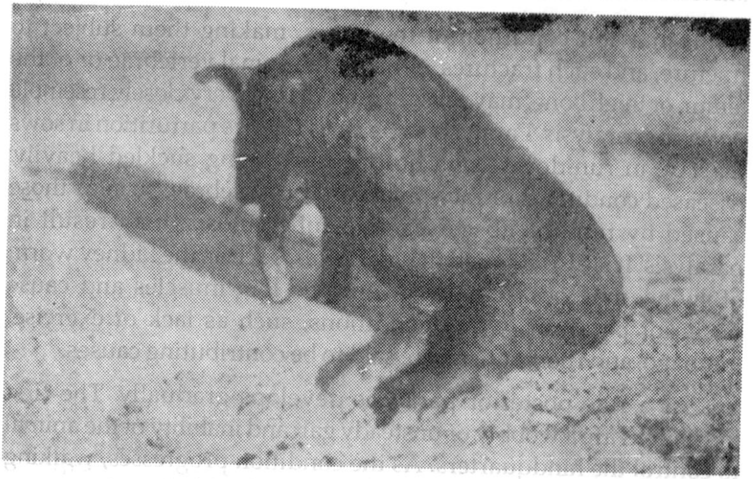

Fig. 2: The posture of this hog is characteristic of the advanced stage of posterior paralysis. (Courtesy of Charles Murray).

In view of the probability that many cases of posterior paralysis are caused by vitamin and mineral deficiencies, preventive measures consist in providing the animals with a well-balanced ration and meeting their mineral requirements. This may be accomplished by adding green feeds to the usual ration, which is often deficient in the essential vitamin A; if green feeds are not available, fish oils may be substituted. Mineral is supplied by adding steamed bonemeal to the diet. As additional preventive measures, care should be taken to prevent injury to the pigs, and they should have plenty of exercise and sunlight, and sanitary surroundings at all times.

Pneumonia

Pneumonia is rather commonly associated with hog cholera, swine plague, and other acute infectious conditions of swine; it is of much less frequent occurrence as a primary or specific disease. When not associated with other diseases, pneumonia probably occurs most frequently in the septic, or gangrenous, form.

Pneumonia always results from some form of irritation of the lung tissue. The nonspecific types may be due to a number of causative factors, such as exposure to severe weather conditions, the inbreathing of dust or other irritating substances, the introduction of foreign material into the lung as a result of improper drenching, and any form of mechanical injury to the lung tissue.

The various forms of irritation mentioned lead to inflammatory changes and consequent solidification of the lung tissue, so that little air space is left in the parts of the lung involved. In the advanced stages the lung becomes hepatized, or liverlike, to such an extent that portions of the affected tissue will sink when placed in water.

The acute pneumonias are attended by chills, elevation of temperature, and difficult and rapid breathing with some evidence of pain. The affected hogs frequently appear to be trying to obtain some relief by lying on the chest. In all acute types of pneumonia there is a similarity of symptoms regardless of the specific causative agent. This may tend to cause some confusion, as in cases of hog cholera and other infectious diseases with which pneumonia may be associated. There are, however, certain differentiating features which should be kept in mind when pneumonia is present in a herd. In the ordinary types of pneumonia–that is, those not associated with some other disease-usually only a few animals in the herd are affected, and their temperature seldom exceeds 104° F. (normal for a hog is 101° F.), whereas when pneumonia accompanies such diseases as hog cholera the temperature is usually several degrees higher, and more animals are sick. The disease runs a milder course in the ordinary types, and many of the animals recover, while in cholera the course of the disease is rapid, and most of the affected animals succumb.

Autopsies on hogs dead from pneumonia commonly reveal the solidification of the lung already mentioned. Sometimes puslike material is present, and there may be centers of dead tissue (necrosis) in the lung. There is an absence of congestion, hemorrhages, and similar lesions in other tissues and organs, where they are found in hog cholera. Pneumonia due to lungworms is chronic in type, and as a rule only certain areas of the lung tissue are involved.

Pneumonia may be prevented to a large extent by correct sanitary measures and proper handling of the herd, particularly under severe weather conditions. The quarters where swine are kept should be reasonably sanitary, protected from cold, and properly ventilated without drafts. Hogs should not be permitted to burrow under straw-stacks where they are crowded together and become overheated; when they come out from such places into the cold at feeding time, they become chilled, and chilling is very conductive to pneumonia. Feeding hogs on clean concrete floors will aid very materially in preventing worm infestations, which may result in verminous pneumonia.

When pneumonia is known to be present in the herd, proper care and handling are of extreme importance in aiding recovery. The sick hogs should be housed in warm, clean, dry quarters where there is proper ventilation without drafts. A box stall is desirable when available. There should be an ample supply of clean drinking water. A purgative such as Epsom salts should be given early in the disease. If the animals show an inclination to eat, give bran mashes or other kinds of soft sloppy feed.

Since pneumonia is frequently associated with certain acute infectious diseases of swine, owners should be on the alert for possible outbreaks of such serious infections as hog cholera when a considerable number of the animals in a herd are observed to be sick. A veterinarian should be consulted immediately with a view to obtaining a prompt and accurate diagnosis, and his advice with regard to the proper procedure in controlling and preventing the further spread of the disease should be strictly followed. Prompt action in such cases may prevent heavy losses in affected herds.

Mastitis (Mammitis, or Garget)

Mastitis, or mammitis, also referred to as garget, is an inflammatory condition of the mammary gland, or udder.

Owing to their location and the conformation of the animal, the mammary glands of swine are predisposed to various kinds of injuries, such as bruises or abrasions from contact with stubble, stones, and other objects. As a result of such injuries, various types of bacteria, particularly pyogenic (pus-producing) organisms, gain entrance to the udder tissues. Organisms may also reach the gland tissues through the teat cavities. The invasion of the infective organisms is followed by inflammation.

The inflamed udder becomes swollen, hot, and paipful. Milk that is forced out of the infected gland is clotted or more or less ropy. As the condition progresses, abscesses may form. In some cases there is a general disturbance of the system, resulting in loss of appetite, rise of temperature, and possibly constipation. Owing to the soreness of the affected udder, the sow frequently will not permit the pigs to nurse.

In cases of acute mammitis, alternate hot and cold applications, when practicable, will prove helpful in reducing the inflammation of the udder. The sow should also be given a purgative, such as Epsom salts. If there are open wounds or sores, they should be thoroughly cleaned with warm water, after which either iodized glycerine or antiseptic dusting powders may be applied. In cases of abscess formation, the condition can be satisfactorily relieved only through surgical means. In addition to the acute, more common, pyogenic form of mammitis in swine there are also several other forms, more chronic in character and due to different types of infection, such as actinomycosis, tuberculosis, and botryomycosis.

Actinomycosis of the udder is caused by the actinomyces, or ray fungus, which is widespread in nature, particularly on grains and grasses. Infection of this type is, therefore, most likely to be observed in the udders of sows that have been pasturing on stubble fields. The infective agent gains entrance to the udder tissue through injuries or abrasions of the skin. The lesions are quite similar in appearance to the changes seen in actinomycosis of other tissues and are characterized by tumefactions, or enlargements, which may vary in size from an inch to several inches in diameter. The enlargements may become eroded and rupture, discharging a sticky, granular, light-yellowish pus. Medicinal agents are of little value as treatment, and usually relief must be obtained by removing the entire tumefaction through proper surgical procedure.

In tuberculous mammitis, caused by the tubercle bacillus, technically called *Mycobacterium tuberculosis*, the lesions, or tissue changes, are the same as those observed in tuberculosis in other parts of the body. In the cases the causative organism may have been introduced from outside sources through injuries, or it may have been transmitted through the circulation from a center of infection in some other tissue or organ. If the tuberculous lesions are localized, or confined to the udder tissue, relief may be obtained by surgical means.

This procedure may be followed when the sow is a valuable animal; otherwise it would be safer to slaughter the animal and cremate the carcass in order to prevent the possible further spread of the infection.

Botryomycotic mammitis, which has been attributed to the presence of *Staphylococcus ascoformans*, is of rare occurrence. The lesions are rather similar in their gross appearance to those of actinomycosis, consisting of fibrous tumorlike enlargements containing numbers of pus centers or cavities. Treatment would consist in surgical removal of the enlargements.

The services of a veterinarian should be obtained for all the conditions in which surgical procedure must be resorted to.

Skin Diseases of Swine

Skin diseases may be classified as parasitic and nonparasitic. Only the latter will be considered here, except in so far as the conditions described may be more or less indirectly the result of parasitic infestation. Diseases and injuries caused by parasites are discussed elsewhere in this volume.

Erythema

Erythema is a reddening of the skin due to congestion of the blood capillaries near the surface, particularly those of the small elevations of the skin or papillae. It may be primary or secondary. The primary type may be the result of various forms of external irritation, including friction, blows, exposure to sunlight, bites by parasites, extreme heat and cold, and chemicals. This type of erythema may also be caused by certain feeds of improper methods of feeding.

The condition is characterized by diffuse reddening of the skin and is, therefore, readily observed only in swine with white or unpigmented skin. The redness disappears on pressure and returns when pressure is removed. The skin feels hot to the touch, and there may be some evidence of pruritis, or itching. Erythema may be the first stage of an inflammatory condition of the skin; otherwise it usually disappears spontaneously after a number of hours, or at most within several days.

Treatment is necessary only when there is considerable itching. Applications of cold water or alcohol give relief. If there is evidence of irritation from rubbing, ordinary dusting powders or zinc ointment may be used. Preventive measures consist in providing proper sanitary conditions, giving careful attention to the feed, and ridding the animals of any lice that may be present.

Erythema occurs as a secondary condition in a number of acute infectious diseases, such as hog cholera, swine plague, and swine erysipelas, and this fact should be kept in mind when the condition is observed in the herd.

Urticaria (Nettle Rash)

Urticaria (called hives in human beings) is a skin affection characterized by slightly raised and reddened areas on the skin surface. Pigs are more frequently affected than mature swine. The condition is thought to be due in many cases to a general disturbance of the system, as in the case of a digestive derangement. Certain feeds–buckwheat, for example–may cause urticaria in older hogs; this is a type of allergy. The condition may also result from external irritations and filthy surroundings.

The reddened areas of the skin are hot, and there is evidence of itching. In these cases, applications of alcohol or cold water have a good effect. A purgative, such as Epsom salts, is in order. With the necessary corrective measure, including proper diet and the removal of irritating factors, the skin lesions usually heal spontaneously without recourse to treatment of any kind.

Eczema

Eczema is observed most frequently in pigs and is comparatively rare in older swine. In this condition there is a definite inflammation of the skin with eruptions on various parts of the body.

Eczema is usually associated with digestive derangement, improper care and feeding, and an insanitary environment. The condition is also seen in pigs that have become weak and emaciated as a result of chronic diseases, such as hog cholera and swine plague. Primary irritation of the skin by lice may also lead to eczema.

Eczema is characterized by erythema, or reddening of the skin, and the formation of small nodules with vesicles, or blisters, and pustules (swellings containing pus). After being ruptured, the vesicles and pustules dry up, forming scabs. At this stage there is intense itching, and as a result of injuries caused by rubbing there may be considerable scaling of the surface layer of skin and consequent inflammatory changes, accompanied by pus, in the deeper skin structures. In the later stages of this conditions the skin may become thickened and hard and show cracks and some bleeding.

Eczema may be differentiated from mange by the absence of parasites. In some cases the eczematous lesions may simulate swine pox, though the skin lesions of the latter are rather characteristic.

Treatment consists largely of preventive measures, such as removing or avoiding all predisposing factors, through providing sanitary surroundings and seeing that pigs have good rations. All pigs affected should have a purgative, such as Epsom salts. Zinc ointment and antiseptic dusting powders may be applied to the skin lesions.

Sunburn and Frostbite

Pigs that have white skin or very little pigment in the skin are susceptible to sunburn on exposure to the direct rays of the sun. At first there will simply be reddening of the skin, but if the exposure is continued a definite dermatitis, or skin inflammation, will develop, with more or less sloughing of the surface layer and eventually thickening and hardening. Pigs so affected do not thrive.

Preventive treatment is self-evident and consists in providing shade to protect the hogs from continued exposure to the direct rays of the sun, particularly during the hot season. Applications of mild antiseptics and ointments would be indicated in cases of considerable destruction of skin tissue.

Pigs farrowed during the cold season, particularly in northern regions, may be frozen when the sows are not properly housed and protected from the cold. The parts most frequently affected are the ears and tail. The frosting of the tissues may result in an inflammatory condition. If the tissues are completely frozen, there will be considerable sloughing of the parts and sometimes the loss of ears and tail.

Occasionally the skin of mature hogs may be frozen as a result of exposure, as during shipping, and this also may result in inflammation and possible sloughing.

Prevention consists in protecting the hogs against extreme weather conditions. Skin lesions caused by freezing may be treated with mild antiseptics and ointments, like similar skin conditions.

Swine Plague (Hemorrhagic Septicemia)

Swine plague, or hemorrhagic septicemia, is an infectious disease of swine caused by a specific organism, *Pasteurella suiseptica.* The organism is rather widespread in nature and may also be found in the air passages and intestinal tracts of apparently normal hogs.

Swine plague apparently occurs rather frequently in its septicemic (blood-poisoning) form in European countries and hence is recognized there as an independent disease, but in the United States it is seen more often as a complication in certain other diseases, particularly hog cholera. Because of this frequent association with other conditions, there has been some question as to whether swine plague does occur in this country as a specific disease. Although further studies will be required to clear up certain points, present information indicates that it probably does occur independently from time to time, particularly as a pulmonary type of infection, or pneumonia, and usually as scattered cases.

It seems evident that *Pasteurella suiseptica*, which ordinarily is harmless, or nonpathogenic, to healthy swine, becomes capable of producing disease under certain conditoins, such as lowered vitality, which make the tissues more susceptible to invasion. The organism may survive for a certain period in insanitary surroundings or in dark places, but it is rather quickly destroyed by sunlight and ordinary disinfectants. The infection is rarely transmitted directly from animal to animal and seldom spreads beyond the herds affected.

A number of factors may result in diminished resistance of swine to hemorrhagic septicemia infection, including exposure to cold, exhaustion from shipping, weaning, poor housing, improper feeding, and different forms of irritation of the lung tissues, as from excessive dust or parasites.

In the uncomplicated form of swine plague, manifested chiefly as pneumonia, the respiratory tract is the channel through which infection commonly takes place. The severity of the symptoms and the extent of the tissue damage depend on the virulence of the infective organisms and the resistance of the individual animals.

The symptoms commonly observed in this country are those usually seen in pneumonia. The temperature may rise to possibly 105° F., and there may be rapid and difficult breathing and a spasmodic cough, with a discharge of mucus or mucus and pus from the mouth and nose. In some cases there is conjunctivitis (inflammation of the mucus membranes of the eyes) and a purulent discharge from the eyes. Other symptoms are partial or complete loss of appetite and constipation, which may be followed by a bloody diarrhoea. Diffuse reddening of the skin may be noticed. In some cases there is a tendency for the affected hog to sit on its haunches. As the disease progresses, extreme weakness and emaciation occur, and breathing becomes difficult. Finally, complete prostration occurs, and death may ensue in from 1 to 2 weeks. Few hogs make a complete recovery. In those surviving, the disease usually assumes a chronic form in which there is continued difficult breathing, a persistent cough, poor appetite, progressive weakness, emaciation, and in some cases a fetid diarrhoea, and after a number of weeks the animals die from exhaustion.

The lesions found on autopsy are chiefly those of pneumonia, or extensive solidification of the lung tissue. The involved tissue may vary from reddish or brown to gray in different portions, and this variation gives the cut surface of the lungs a mottled appearance. Dead areas of lung tissue (necrosis) will be seen, their extent depending somewhat on the length of time the pneumonia has been present. Inflammatory changes in the pleura, or thin membrane covering the lungs, together with a purulent condition, may be seen in some cases. The lymph glands associated with the lungs (the bronchial and mediastinal glands) will be hemorrhagic, and in the more chronic cases may contain centers of dead tissue.

Diagnosis and Control Measures

The problem of reaching a definite diagnosis of swine plague is greatly complicated by the fact that it is so frequently associated with hog cholera. It is impossible through observation, for even an experienced veterinarian to differentiate between the two diseases in herds where there is possibility of the presence of hog cholera. In such cases a definite diagnosis can be made only by demonstrating that the causative organism of swine plague is in the blood or tissues of the affected hogs, and by determining the presence of the virus of hog cholera through swine inoculations with filtered blood from the affected hog. It may also be difficult to differentiate in some cases between pneumonia due to swine plague and some of the more common types of pneumonia in swine.

No specific curative treatment for the disease is known. There are hemorrhagic septicemia serums, aggressins, and bacterins on the market which have been used to some advantage, particularly as preventive agents. The most effective means of prevention, however, consists in practicing proper sanitation. Hog houses and their surroundings should be kept in a reasonably sanitary condition at all times. Since dusty pens in dry weather tend to favour infection, wetting grounds and floors with water or a weak disinfectant from time to time is a helpful preventive measure. Hogs should be properly housed and protected against severe weather conditions during the winter. Treatment of the sick animals is largely a matter of proper care and handling. Sick hogs should be removed from the herd and placed in clean, dry quarters with plenty of fresh air but without drafts. Plenty of clean drinking water should always be available. The feed should be of a soft, sloppy nature and limited in amount until the animals show improved appetite. Recovery is usually slow, and because of the tendency of the disease to become chronic and the continued emaciation and lack of vitality of the affected animals, they may become a total loss to the owner.

When swine plague occurs as a complication of hog cholera, the sick animals should be handled and treated as they would be for the latter disease alone. Under such circumstances it is advisable to consult a veterinarian immediately and follows his recommendations.

Chapter 6

BRUCELLOSIS (INFECTIOUS ABORTION) IN SWINE

Adolph Eichhorn[1]

[1] *Adolph Eichhorn is Director, Animal Disease Station, Bureau of Animal Industry.*

Fewer swine than cattle get brucellosis, but on the other hand half the cases of undulant fever in human beings are due to infection with the swine organism; and the latter also causes a more severe disease in human beings than the cattle organism. Systematic eradication of swine brucellosis, then, is a matter of considerable importance in the public interest.

Following the epoch-making discovery by the Danish investigator, Bang, in 1896, that abortion in cattle may be induced by the micro-organism *Brucella abortus*, the disease, then called contagious abortion, was also found to be present in cattle in the United States. It was not until 1914, however, that a similar disease in swine was reported by Traum, who recovered from the aborted fetuses of a sow an organism similar to that causing abortions in cattle.

Subsequent investigations showed that the organism infecting swine was slightly different from the cattle type. A third type was recovered from goats affected with a similar disease. Therefore the generic name *Brucella* was given to these three closely related germs, the cattle species being called *Br. abortus*, the swine species, *Br. suis*, and the goat species, *Br. melitensis*. The medical term "brucellosis" has been given to the diseases in all animals caused by any and all of the three *Brucella* organisms. More popularly, the three diseases are known respectively as Bang's disease, contagious abortion of swine, and Malta fever of goats.

From recent surveys brucellosis in swine appears to be much more restricted than brucellosis in cattle, the latter unquestionably being one of the most important diseases affecting the cattle industry. The swine disease, however, may become a very serious menace, not only to the swine industry but also to public health, as will be shown later, unless definite, systematic measures of control or eradication are instituted.

Since Traum's discovery of brucellosis in swine, investigations of the disease have been made by the Bureau of Animal Industry and other research institutions in the United States and foreign countries. In 1922 Schroeder showed that the swine species of the *Brucella* organism possesses greater virulence for guinea pigs than the bovine species of *Brucella*. Subsequent investigations conducted by Schroeder and Cotton, Buck, and others in the United States have shown that cattle thoroughly exposed to infected swine do not contract the disease and develop only a temporary reaction to the blood-agglutination test used to detect the presence of the disease.

While some investigators report that as many as 20 percent of all sows are infected, a more careful survey in Iowa showed that only 2.5 percent in that State reacted to the agglutination test. In other localities in the Middle West approximately the same percentage of infection in hogs as in Iowa, or a lower one, was found.

The disease is usually introduced into a herd through the purchase of an infected animal and may be spread through the ingestion by the animals of aborted fetuses and fetal membranes, as well as through contaminated food and drinking water. Infection through the skin and membranes of the eye might also occur in some instances. The possibility of transmission of the disease from cattle to swine through the eating of aborted cattle fetuses and membranes has been suggested, but experimental evidence shows that swine are extremely resistant to the bovine species of *Brucella*.

Lesions

Following infection, the germs of the disease are usually present in the blood, through which they reach the lymph glands, spleen, udder, and bones, causing inflammatory conditions at the points of localization. In the male animals the infection frequently causes a severe destructive inflammation of the testicles and seminal vesicles, which results in a marked swelling of the testes and the epididymis-the tubes at the back of the testes–and may affect the general condition of the animal. Boars so affected are frequently defective in breeding capacity, and the infection may result in impotency if both testicles are affected.

As each fetus in the sow is enveloped in a separate membrane, it is not uncommon for some fetuses in a litter to be born fully developed, while others show that death occurred prior to the termination of pregnancy. Most often the fetuses die following the act of abortion, though mummified fetuses are not infrequent, especially when the fetus has died a considerable time before abortion took place. In cases of abortion, the membranes of the sow disclose hemorrhages, and there is a grayish-brown exudate, or discharge similar to that observed in the disease in cattle.

Not infrequently the disease is associated with arthritis, resulting in suppuration (generation of pus) at a joint and erosion, or slow destruction of the cartilage. Abscess formations may be observed in the liver, spleen, and other parts of the body. The bones of the spinal column may become affected, and abscesses may develop which in advanced cases are enclosed in a capsule of connective tissue. These changes may become aggravated and result in deformity of the spine and impairment of locomotion.

Symptoms

The symptoms are not unlike those occurring in cattle. A day before abortion, there is swelling of the udder and vulva, and milk makes its appearance in the teats. At times the sow shows illness prior to abortion, lying down a great deal of the time and at other times being restless and uneasy, and not infrequently develops a discharge from the vagina. There is rarely any discharge after abortion, except that when abortion occurs during the early stages of pregnancy there may be a dark-grayish discharge several days afterward. The expulsion of the fetus takes some time, and there is no indication of labour pains. The fetuses are expelled in the enveloping membranes and hence there is no retained placenta, or after birth, as is often the case in aborting cows. In some instances inflammation of the uterus follows, but usually the sow makes a rapid recovery. The sow usually comes in heat within a few days after abortion, but as a rule several negative breedings take place before she again becomes pregnant. Animals that have aborted once do not usually do so again. The time of the occurrence of abortion varies considerably and is unquestionably dependent on the time and the virulence of infection, but usually it takes place between the sixtieth and ninetieth days of pregnancy.

Diagnosis

It is very essential to examine the boars carefully in all instances of abortion among swine. Diagnosis is made by isolating the *Brucella* organism from the infected animals and also by the agglutination test. Since the organism grows readily on artificial culture media, its isolation is not difficult. The infection is most frequently found in the genitals of reacting boars and in the stomach contents of aborted fetuses. *Br. suis* is often present in pure culture and may be readily identified by appropriate procedures.

Abortions caused by brucellosis should not be confused with abortions from other causes. Mechanical injuries to the sow, the presence of other infections, and vitamin or mineral deficiencies also may cause abortion. It is essential, therefore, to confirm the diagnosis by the isolation of the organism or by positive blood tests. The blood test is unquestionably the most readily available diagnostic method, but it apparently is not as reliable as the test in cattle.[2] Experiments to establish whether an antigen, or testing agent, produced from swine strains is more reliable than that prepared from bovine strains have not shown any advantage for the former, and therefore the antigen generally employed for testing is prepared from a bovine strain. Other biological tests have been used for the diagnosis of the disease in swine, but they have failed to show any superiority over the agglutination test, or even as much accuracy.

Prevention and Control

There is no specific drug or other chemical agent known for the cure of the infection. As in the case of bovine abortion, various

---

[2] Agglutination in dilutions of 1 to 50 or higher is indicative of infection, and agglutination of 1 to 25 should be considered suspicious. Not infrequently the agglutination test shows no reaction until after the animal has aborted. For details of the test and its interpretation, the reader is referred to Farmers' Bulletin 1871, Brucellosis of Cattle.

remedies for the prevention and treatment of the disease are being exploited, but in all instances they have failed to show any merit. Attention must therefore be directed toward prevention of the disease. Where the infection is suspected, all animals should be subjected to the blood test. Like brucellosis in cattle, the disease in swine tends to be self-limiting. Animals that have aborted may become immune, or even if they should harbour the infection they carry their fetuses through the normal period of pregnancy. It is advisable, however, after the presence of the infection has been established, to eliminate all reacting animals and subject the rest of the herd to frequent blood tests until there is no evidence of a suspicious or reacting animal. This should be accompanied by adequate sanitary measures.

In its resistance to physical and chemical exposure, *Brucella suis* behaves like the organism of the bovine type. Thus, the article in this book dealing with the disease in cattle should be carefully studied and the sanitary measures recommended for its control should be applied to the elimination of the infection in swine.

While calfhood vaccination for the control of the disease in cattle has given very encouraging results, few experimental data are available on the immunization of swine. In Isolated instances cultures prepared from strain 19, used in calf vaccination, have been employed for immunization in swine, but no data are available as to their efficacy. Experimental work is still in progress.

Public Health Hazard

From a public health standpoint, human infection with the swine type of *Brucella* is unquestionably more important than human infection with the bovine type. It is a recognized fact that *Brucella melitensis*, the goat type, induces the most severe type of undulant fever, the disease in human beings. Next in order is the swine type, and last, the bovine type. This fact has been established by isolating the various types of organisms from infected human beings and observing the severity of the disease caused by each of the three species. It has been estimated by Public Health Service officials that about 50 percent of human infection is due to *Br. suis* and is the result of contact with infected swine on farms or in abattoirs. The frequent occurrence of the disease in human beings in swine-raising localities is indicative of the danger, and the disease often occurs among workers in packing houses as a result of handling carcasses of infected swine. Studies have shown that in the Corn Belt more than half the cases of undulant fever are caused by the swine type and that in regions where the infection in hogs is not common this type of infection in man is less frequent.

Chapter 7

MANGE OF SWINE

Marion Imes[1]

[1] *Marion Imes is Senior Veterinarian, Zoological Division, Bureau of Animal Industry.*

A suitable dip, used in a vat or a hog wallow, will get rid of common mange of hogs. The method of treatment is described here, and it is worth putting into practice because when mange takes hold it can be very expensive to the hog owner.

Common mange of hogs is a contagious skin disease which costs swine growers huge sums of money each year, and they pay the bill whether they know it or not. There are no specific data on losses at the farm and feed lot, but as mange stunts the growth of young hogs, delays fattening, and causes some deaths, the estimated losses at these sources probably average about $2 an animal in infected herds. In addition, mangy hogs shipped to market are usually sold at a discount of from 50 cents to $1.50 a hundred weight. The average yield of the principal cuts per hog at packing houses is 35 pounds of hams, 30 pounds of bacon, and 15 pounds of picnics, or a total of 80 pounds of the most valuable parts of the carcass. When the skin over these parts is mangy, the grade and consequently the selling price are lowered–hence the discount on the price of the live hog.

Common mange is more or less prevalent throughout the United States, and the total number of infected hogs is large. The losses, therefore, are sufficiently impressive to emphasize the fact that the disease is a serious menace to the industry. Fortunately there is a brighter side to the picture. Several years ago the Bureau of Animal Industry made an investigation of mange of swine and conducted experiments on treating infected hogs, and the findings showed that the disease yields readily to proper treatment and is easily eradicated.

A contagious disease, however, cannot be eradicated by temporizing or following slipshod methods. Mange is caused by a well-known parasite and is not a filth-borne disease. Good sanitation and careful feeding are essential parts of all successful methods of swine production, but shifting undipped hogs to clean lots, changing or increasing the feed or adding medicines to it, sprinkling dry lime-sulfur in the bedding, or hand treating only the well-developed skin lesions will not eradicate hog mange.

Swine in the United States are affected by two kinds of mange, sarcoptic and demodectic, caused by two different genera of mites–*Sarcoptes* and *Demodex*–which live in the skin of the host animal.

The entire life cylces of the mites are passed on the host animal. In obtaining their food from the tissues and blood and preparing suitable places for their various life processes, the mites cause characteristic wounds, or lesions, in the skin. The sarcoptic mites burrow into the skin, each female making a separate gallery in which she lays her eggs. The skin over and around the burrows becomes inflamed, and small vesicles and cone-shaped swellings appear. The demodectic mites, which cause demodectic, or follicular, mange, live in colonies or groups in the hair follicles and sebaceous glands and cause small hard swellings or pimples.

Sarcoptic Mange

Sarcoptic, or common, mange occurs in all parts of the United States where hogs are raised. Traffic in breeding stock evidently has been an important factor in spreading the disease. Under conditions favourable to it, mange spreads rapidly unless active measures are taken to control it. Hogs of all classes and ages are susceptible to the infection, but young stock and poorly nourished, older animals of low vitality suffer most.

The mites that cause sarcoptic mange of swine are known as *Sarcoptes scabiei suis*. These mites are small white or yellowish insectlike parasites, visible to the naked eye, especially when they are placed against a dark background. The mature female is about one-fiftieth and the male is about one-sixtieth of an inch in length. They are plainly visible under an ordinary hand lens.

The general form of the body is round, and the bluntly rounded head is as broad as it is long. The mature mites have four pairs of short thick legs, the fourth pair and usually the third pair not extending beyond the margin of the body. Under a high-power microscope a number of short, backward-projecting spines can be seen on the upper surface of the body.

In the burrows or galleries made by the mites in the skin each female may lay from 10 to 25 eggs, which hatch in 3 to 10 days. The mites of the new generation form new burrows and begin laying eggs when they are 10 to 12 days old. The average period of incubation is about 4 days and the average period between hatching and egg laying about 11 days.

Symptoms

The first lesions of sarcoptic mange usually appear on the head of a hog, around the eyes, nose, or ears, where the skin is tender and the hair is thin. From these parts the infection spreads over the neck, shoulders, and back and along the sides, finally involving the entire body. The mites cause irritation, itching, inflammation, and swelling in the sensitive tissues of the skin. Nodules and vesicles appear over and around the burrows. The vesicles break and discharge serum, which usually dries into hard granules or scales. The hair over the lesions stands erect, and some of it drops out.

As the mites multiply and the disease advances increasingly large areas of skin become involved. The nodules increase in number and are closer together. The mechanical injury to the skin resulting from rubbing and other efforts to relieve the intense itching cause large scabs that may be stained yellowish or reddish by serum or blood. The skin becomes thickened and is thrown into wrinkles or folds. Scrapings taken from moist furrows of the wrinkles usually contain mites. In chronic cases of the moist form of the disease there is a very offensive odor. When the mites are not very active, the surface of the affected skin may be a silver-gray colour and have a dry, scurfy, or leatherlike appearance. In such cases the mites are difficult to find.

Positive diagnosis consists in finding the mites, which are the sole cause of the disease, but on account of their burrowing habit this is not always easy. They may be found by deeply scraping the affected area with a blunt-edged knife and examining the scrapings in warm sunshine or near artificial heat, under a low-power magnifying glass. Well-advanced cases of mange are easy to detect, but since the disease should not be allowed to reach this stage, early diagnosis is important. Repeated rubbing, scratching, or biting in one place indicates irritation and itching and should be investigated at once by a close examination of the animal. Disarranged hair indicates the area of skin to be examined. If the skin is thickened and hardened and dried serum or scabs are present, search should be made for mange mites.

Contagiousness

Sarcoptic mange is contagious to all animals of the same species. It is transmissible from one species of animal to another, and in some cases from animals to man. Sarcoptic mites of the hog are knows to be transmissible to man. They live only a limited time on the human host but may produce lesions that persist for 30 days or longer and cause extreme annoyance. It is advisable, therefore, to change clothes and bathe after handling mangy hogs.

The disease is usually transmitted among swine by direct contact of uninfected with infected animals, but it may be contracted from infected enclosures, equipment used on or around infected animals, or other objects that are carriers of the mites. Although they cannot propagate except on the host animal, dislodged mites that drop in moist shady places may retain their vitality for 4 weeks or longer during mild weather. Bright sunshine, freezing weather, and lack of moisture usually destroy mites and eggs not on an animal in a few days.

Usually the disease spreads slowly during warm weather, especially when the animals are on pasture, but it spreads rapidly when hogs are closely confined in small enclosures. Exposure to inclement weather, insufficient feed or feed of poor quality, or any other circumstance tending to lessen the vitality or functional activities of the hogs hastens the spread and development of mange. When the mites are active and new lesions are developing, the entire body surface may become involved in about 6 weeks.

Attacks of the disease do not confer immunity, and hogs may become infected any number of times. Since sarcoptic mange is contagious, plans for keeping hogs free from the disease should include precautionary measures against the introduction of infection by such means as bringing undipped animals onto the premises, contact between clean and infected hogs separated only by a wire fence, and allowing hogs to occupy infected premises.

All small enclosures that have been occupied by infected hogs should be cleaned and disinfected before they are used for healthy hogs. Remove all litter, cleaning down to a smooth surface, then spray the exposed surfaces with coal-tar-creosote dip or disinfectant diluted in accordance with the directions on the label of the container. The coal-tar-creosote preparations are sold under many different trade names, and when properly diluted with water they are suitable for use as disinfectants on animals as well as for premises.

Treatment

The proper treatment of hogs infected with sarcoptic mange mites consists in killing the parasites without injuring the animals by applying medicated liquids known as dips. Of the several different kinds of effective dips available, oils and lime-sulfur are the ones most commonly and successfully used. These are obtainable ready-prepared for dilution with water, or they may be made by the user. Ready-prepared dips should be diluted and used in accordance with the instructions on the label.

In treating hogs for mange the entire herd should be treated regardless of the number showing visible lesions. To select and treat only those with well-advanced cases of mange will not eradicate the disease, as any member of the herd may at any time carry the parasites temporarily without showing visible lesions. In some cases the disease may be dormant during the summer and early fall months, but with the advent of cold inclement weather it may develop very rapidly. When the weather is too cold for dipping or other effective treatment, rapid spread of the disease may be checked temporarily by hand applications of dips to the worst cases, but mange cannot be eradicated by such methods. Dipping during the mild weather of autumn is good insurance against the risk of loss from mange and the probable additional expense of winter treatment.

Sows heavy with young should not be dipped or oiled within 2 weeks of their farrowing time or too soon after farrowing. When the pigs are 3 weeks old, the sow and pigs may be dipped or treated without undue risk of injury. All the pigs of the litter should be dipped or treated in the same manner as the sow; otherwise she may fail to recognize and to suckle some of them. As mange affects the heads and ears of hogs, it is necessary to submerge, or duck, the head of each hog as it swims through the dip.

Dips

The most effective known dip for sarcoptic or common mange of hogs is crude petroleum or some of the oils derived from it. Unprocessed crude oil is often difficult to obtain and is more expensive than some of the processed oils. The various processed oils vary greatly in the number and relative percentages of their constituents, and there is no fixed standard for oil dips for hogs. The processed oils from which the gasoline and other light hydrocarbons have been removed are usually suitable, but those from which the lubricating oils have been removed are not.

Used lubricating oils, drained from the crankcases of automobiles and other engines, are suitable and effective as dips for hogs, but lubricating oil is not suitable for use on cattle, horses, or sheep. When properly used on hogs, lubricating oil is an effective remedy for mange, it does not injure the animals, and it is usually available at low cost. Several proprietary brands of oil dips are available and are usually effective, but they cost more than crankcase drainings.

In preparing an oil dip, fill the vat with water to within about 6 or 8 inches of the dip line (40 to 48 inches from the bottom) and add sufficient oil to bring the fluid up to that line. The oil floats on the water, forming a layer 6 to 8 inches deep, depending on the quantity added, and as the hogs swim through the vat their bodies become coated with oil. It is not necessary to retard the progress of the animals through the vat. Oil dips are used cold, and one dipping is usually sufficient to eradicate ordinary mange. Hogs with thick adherent scabs from old chronic infections should be dipped two or more times. The proper interval between dippings in oil is about 10 days.

Shade or shelter should be provided for freshly oiled hogs, which should not be exposed to bright, hot sunshine or cold, inclement weather for 24 hours or longer after being oiled. Injury may result also from too much exercise or overheating if the freshly oiled animals are moved rapidly or driven too far.

Lime-sulfur dip is effective in eradicating common mange of hogs when four or more dippings are given at intervals of 6 or 7 days. The temperature of the dip while the animals are in it should be maintained at 95° to 100° F., and visibly infected hogs should be held in the swim 3 minutes. Scrubbing and soaking any lesions covered by hard scabs with warm dip just before the first dipping is recommended.

Proprietary brands of lime-sulfur dip, in the form of concentrated liquid, powder, or crystals, the latter two known as dry lime-sulfur, are available. These products are standardized and are equal to or even better than home-made lime-sulfur dip. Unless the user has proper equipment for preparing the home-made product, the prepared dips are also cheaper.

Methods of Applying Dips

A properly constructed dipping vat or hog wallow[2] is necessary for the proper treatment of any considerable number of hogs. Hog-dipping vats made of galvanized iron, ready for setting in the ground, may be purchased, or vats made of concrete or wood may be constructed on the premises. They are usually arranged so that the hogs enter one end of the vat filled with dip, swim through, and leave the vat at the opposite end, where they enter a draining pen with a watertight sloping floor from which the surplus dip that drips from them flows back into the vat.

The liquid in the vat should be from 40 to 48 inches deep, which is sufficient to swim the tallest animal. A full-grown hog carries out of the vat and retains on an average about 1 quart of dip, and the average quantity for each animal of a mixed herd is about 1½ pints. Adding the quantity of dip carried out and retained by the hogs to the quantity required to charge the vat originally gives the approximate quantity needed to complete the dipping process for a given herd. The capacity of the vat in gallons is obtained by

---

[2] IMES, MARION, HOG LICE AND HOG MANGE: METHODS OF CONTROL AND ERADICATION, U.S. Dept. Agr. Farmers' Bul. 1085, 28 pp., illus. 1920. (Revised, 1937).

multiplying the average length in inches by the average depth, then the product by the average width, and dividing by 231, the number of cubic inches in a gallon. The average length of a vat with sloping sides is obtained by adding the length in inches at the dip line to the length at the bottom and dividing by 2, and the average width in a similar manner.

If shallow water is available, hogs will wallow in it when the weather is warm, and this habit may be utilized in preventing or curing mange. Adding oil to the water in properly constructed wallows is an inexpensive and satisfactory method of applying oil to hogs.

The water in the wallow should be about 3 inches deep without oil until the hogs become accustomed to using it. Hogs will not wallow in deep water, and when they lie down in wallows they displace a volume of the liquid, which causes the water line to rise. If they cannot easily keep their nostrils above the liquid, they leave the wallow before their bodies are wet on both sides. After the habit of using the wallow is well fixed, oil may be added and the depth of the liquid increased to 5 or 6 inches, depending on the size of the hogs and as observation and experience may indicate. After the bodies of the animals are well coated with oil, the wallow should be drained, cleaned, and recharged with water only. Oil may be added every 10 days until the desired results are obtained.

Demodectic Mange

The mite known scientifically as *Demodex phylloides*, which is the primary cause of demodectic or follicular mange in hogs, is a minute, wormlike parasite that penetrates into the hair follicles and sebaceous glands of the skin. The mites are microscopic in size, the mature female measuring about one one-hundredth of an inch in length. Positive diagnosis of the disease can be made only by demonstrating the presence of the mites. If the contents of demodex nodules are examined under a microscope, the small wormlike mites are easily identified.

In small numbers demodectic mites apparently do not cause lesions. Although it is difficult to transmit the disease by artificial means, it is classed as contagious. Demodectic mange may spread rapidly on a hog, but the transmission of the disease from one hog to another is usually much slower than the transmission of common or sarcoptic, mange. Ordinarily the disease does not spread to all members of a herd, since many animals are apparently immune, or at least do not contract the disease.

The lesions of demodectic mange appear as small hard nodules, or pimples, in the skin, usually around the eyes or snout, and spread slowly over the under side of the neck, breast, and abdomen, and between the hind legs. The nodules range in size from that of a pinhead to that of a hazelnut and usually contain it material of creamy white colour and cheesy consistence. In advanced cases the nodules may rupture and discharge their contents over the hair and skin, and in rare cases suppurating (pus-generating) cavities result.

There is no known practical cure for demodectic mange in hogs, as the cost of treatment is out of proportion to the usual value of the animals. Individual animals that show lesions of demodectic mange should be removed from the herd and disposed of or killed. The rest of the herd should be dipped in oil or coal-tar-creosote dip and the premises cleaned and disinfected in the same manner as for sarcoptic mange.

Chapter 8

HOG LICE

O.G. Babcock & E.C. Cushing[1]

[1] *O.G. Babcock is Associate Entomologist and E.C. Cushing is Principal Entomologist, Division of Insects Affecting Man and Animals, Bureau of Entomology and Plant Quarantine.*

Why let hogs be tortured by the biggest of all the lice that infest our domestic animals? The remedies are simple, inexpensive, and effective.

Hog lice are so common that they are often considered as one of the evils that must be endured. These bloodsucking insect parasites, however, are so easily controlled that there is little excuse for letting hogs suffer from the constant irritation they cause, or for the owner to put up with the losses they occasion. Generally these losses are so gradual and continuous that the owner is not aware of them and therefore makes no attempt to keep his animals free of the pests. The injury in heavily infested herds is considerable but it can be eliminated by using a few simple and inexpensive control measures. If young pigs that become infested with lice from their mother are allowed to go untreated until they are old enough to market, there may be a reduction in value of 2 to 6 percent.

The presence of hog lice is easily detected, as this is the largest louse commonly infesting domestic animals in the United States. The adult female is about one-fourth inch long and the male a little shorter. Both sexes are of a grayish colour but appear darker on the darker skinned breeds of hogs.

The lice feed frequently and puncture the skin in a different place at each feeding. An animal on which there are only a few of the parasites may be seen to rub and scratch itself on the sides of the pen or on posts, troughs, and other objects. When there is a heavy infestation hogs suffer constant irritation; they are restless and do not eat properly. Ultimately an unthrifty condition results which is sometimes followed by the attacks of other parasites. The constant rubbing and scratching produces sores that do not heal because the lice congregate around the raw tissues and keep them irritated. In the screwworm area these wounds attract screwworms and quickly become infested.

How Hog Lice Breed

Hog lice are parasitic on swine only and spend their entire life on the host. Other animals and even human beings may occasionally transport the insects accidentally from one place to another.

The female deposits the yellowish-white eggs on the bristles of the hog-from 1 to 20 on a bristle–in such places as back of the ears, on the shoulders and neck, and on the flanks. Each mass of eggs is laid within a few seconds, and as many as 90 eggs may be laid by a single female over a 25-day period. Hatching takes place in 12 to 20 days, the eggs at the greatest distance from the body, that is, farthest up the bristles, usually requiring the longest time, especially in cold weather. After emerging from the egg, the transparent young louse becomes fairly active. It seeks the tender skin surface nearest the place where the egg was laid and begins feeding. On hogs that have been heavily infested for some time these tender skin patches become rough and encrusted with scales, beneath which the young lice hide, seeking protection from cold or from extreme heat. Young lice also seek the protection and warmth afforded by the axilla, or hollow between the leg and the body, and the internal parts of the ears. The newly hatched lice become sexually mature in about 10 days, and egg laying may begin on the twelfth day after hatching.

Practically all new infestations occur when the sexually mature females leave the tips of the bristles of their host and attach themselves to the hairs of other hogs with which the host comes in contact. When separated from an animal, hog lice live only 2 or 3 days. Therefore, reasonably clean pens, corrals, and premises which have not held animals for several days are not sources of infestation even though infested hogs may have occupied them previously.

Control Measures

The methods for keeping hogs free of lice are economical and easily applied, and they should be used by every hog owner, whether he raises hogs for market or for home consumption. Two of the simplest remedies are crude petroleum in dipping vats and kerosene-oil emulsion applied by hand. Both are effective in killing hog lice and their eggs. Arsenical dips, coal-tar-creosote emulsions, and lime-sulfur dips have certain disadvantages that make them inferior to kerosene emulsion or crude petroleum for this purpose.

Crude petroleum is the most widely used and satisfactory remedy. Unprocessed crude petroleum, the natural crude oil that has not been subjected to any manufacturing process, is probably the most effective, but processed crude petroleum–the residue from the crude oil after the distillation of gasoline and other light hydrocarbons–can be used as a dip and is very effective in eradicating hog lice as well as mange. Processed crude oils vary greatly in the number and relative percentages of their constituents and consequently in their consistence, or thickness. As a rule, the thinner the processed crude oil is, the better it is as a dip for hogs. The thick, heavy residue left after the extraction of the lubricating oils is not suitable.

Small quantities of distillate are sometimes added to the processed crude oil, and the product is sold at a high price as a special oil having a high degree of efficacy in eradicating hog lice and mange. The effectiveness of the processed oil for mange is increased by adding distillate or kerosene in the proportion of 1 gallon to each 10 gallons of the oil. Heavy processed oils should be diluted with distillate until they flow freely from the container at the usual dipping temperature, but the maximum quantity of distillate added should not exceed 20 percent. There are also several proprietary brands of crude-petroleum dip, consisting of processed crude oil to which other ingredients have been added. They are usually effective, but they cost more than the unmedicated crude oil.

Kerosene emulsion may be prepared as follows: Slice and dissolve ½ pound of soap in 1 gallon of water, heating the water until the soap is dissolved. Add 2 gallons of kerosene, churning or agitating the mixture thoroughly until no free kerosene is observed on top of the liquid. This stock solution is then diluted with 11 gallons of soft water to make about a 15-percent emulsion, which will kill hog lice and their eggs if properly applied to the animals. Kerosene emulsion is not recommended for use in dipping vats or hog wallows.

Dipping and Treating

Dipping hogs in especially designed hog-dipping vats is the most effective and economical means of controlling lice when the number of animals is sufficiently large to warrant the construction of a vat. Using a concrete hog wallow (Fig. 1) is the next most desirable method of treating large numbers of louse-infested animals. Crude petroleum is the preferred material for use in both vats and wallows.

When the size of hogs using the same wallow varies, the most desirable depth of liquid is 3 to 4 inches. About 1 pint of oil is added to the water in the wallow for each pig and 1 quart for each hog. Usually all hogs will have received sufficient treatment in 24 to 48 hours, after which time the wallow should be drained and charged with fresh water. Arsenical dip is dangerous to use in wallows.

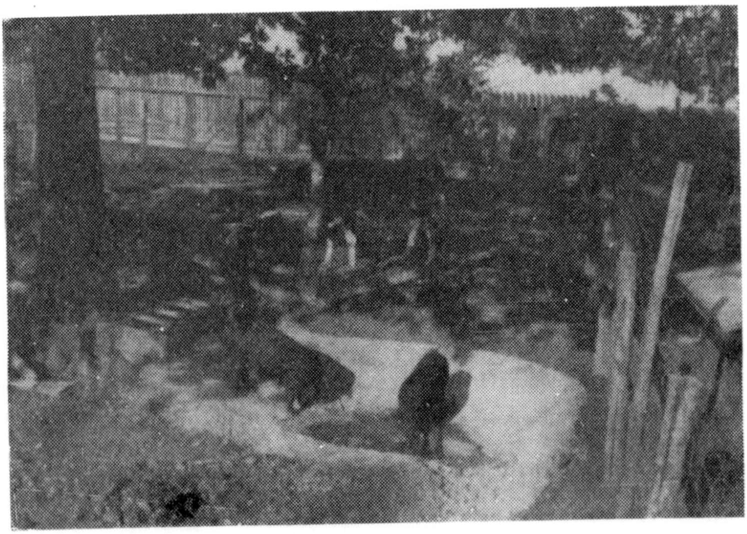

Fig. 1: Small home-made concrete hog wallow.

Complete instructions and specifications for buildings vats and wallows and using crude oil in them are given in Farmers' Bulletin 1085.[2] Anyone contemplating the treatment of hogs by either of these methods should obtain a copy of this publication.

When only a few hogs are to be treated, crude petroleum or kerosene emulsion can be applied by hand. Care should be taken to distribute the insecticide evenly over the entire surface of the head and body of the animal, particular attention being given to the inner surfaces of the ears and to the axillae. The materials can be applied with a brush, mop, or cloth.

Animals should not be treated when they are overheated; and freshly oiled hogs, regardless of the method by which the oil has been applied, should not be forced to move rapidly, or be exposed to bright sunshine, or be allowed to become chilled. The animals should be provided with plenty of shade and moved as little as possible for 24 to 48 hours after treatment, depending on temperature. Apparently oil does not injure hogs if proper care is given them, but this is not true of all species of domestic animals.

Rubbing posts and patented hog oilers have been devised that deposit a small amount of oil on a part of the skin surface when the animal rubs against them. These devices are useful for keeping louse infestations in check, but since only a small part of each animal's body is treated at one time, they cannot be depended on to eradicate lice from a herd. Thorough hand treatment and the use of dipping vats or medicated wallows are the only methods that will give complete control.

---

[2] IMES, MARION. HOG LICE AND HOG MANGE: METHODS OF CONTROL AND ERADICATION. U.S. Dept. Agr. Farmers' Bul. 1085. 22 pp., illus. 1937. (Revised).

Chapter 9

INTERNAL PARASITES OF SWINE

L.A. Spindler[1]

[1] *L A. Spindler is Zoologist, Zoological Division, Bureau of Animal Industry.*

This article discusses all the principal internal parasites of swine in considerable detail, including the damage they do, their life histories, and their relative importance. In equal detail, it outlines systems of control based on careful scientific investigations and shows the great saving that can be made by good management practices.

In the course of centuries swine have come to be afflicted with an imposing array of internal parasites. In the United States they cause extensive losses every year. Like a "fifth column," the parasites seldom give warning of their presence but attack from within, sapping the strength of the host that nourishes and protects them. In general, parasites may have little effect on mature swine, but in young animals they can cause serious injuries. By the time their presence is suspected, they may have undermined the health of the host to such an extent, by imposing a continuous drain on its vitality and sapping its strength little by little, that it never fully recovers, is incapable of normal growth, and makes no profit for the owner.

The extent to which parasites may undermine the health of pigs is illustrated in Figs. 1, *A* & *B*. Pigs farrowed and kept in

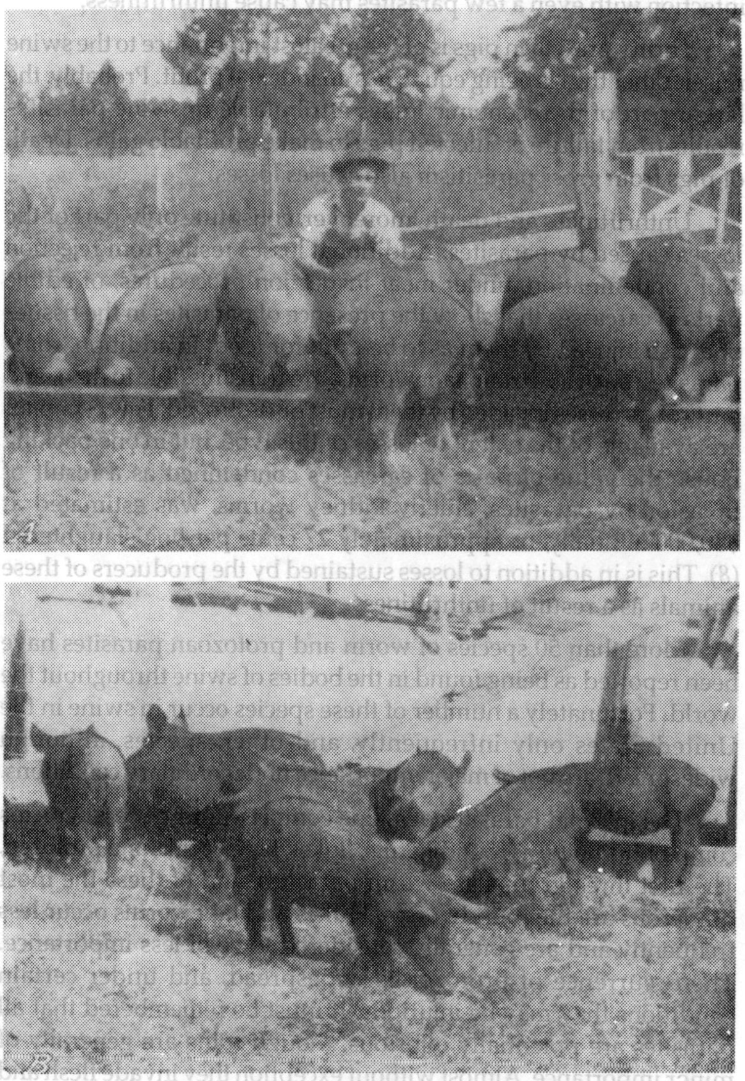

Fig. 1: *A*: These large, healthy pigs were protected from the ravages of parasites; *B*: these unthrifty pigs became parasitized soon after they were born.

permanent, insanitary hog lots may be invaded by parasites even during the first few days of their existence (*21*)[2], and at that age infection with even a few parasites may cause unthriftiness.

Thrifty growth in pigs is of the greatest importance to the swine raiser; other things being equal, it is an index of profit. Probably. the larger part of the economic losses attributable to swine parasites results from failure of infected pigs to make profitable gains. Death of pigs from gross parasitism also causes losses.

Unthriftiness and death, moreover, constitute only part of the losses caused by parasites. Additional losses result from rejection and condemnation, under meat-inspection procedures, of edible parts of carcasses that show the presence of parasites in the tissues or are so injured by them as to be unfit for food. In addition, some parasites, such as certain tapeworms, are transmissible to man, and parts of carcasses invaded by them must be destroyed. Few estimates are available of the extent of losses of this type, but in one packing house the value of parts of carcasses condemned as a result of invasion by parasites, chiefly kidney worms, was estimated at $80,000 annually, or approximately 27 cents per hog slaughtered (*8*). This is in addition to losses sustained by the producers of these animals as a result of unthriftiness.

More than 50 species of worm and protozoan parasites have been reported as being found in the bodies of swine throughout the world. Fortunately a number of these species occur in swine in the United States only infrequently, and other, species, although widespread, are not of major importance under ordinary conditions.

The internal parasites of swine comprise four general groups commonly known as roundworms, flukes, tapeworms, and protozoa, The first three groups are worm parasites, and of these the most numerous are the roundworms. Flukes and tapeworms occur less frequently and are generally considered to be of less importance. The occurrence of protozoa is widespread, and under certain conditions they may be injurious. It must be remembered that all parasites are potentially injurious, though some are generally of minor importance. Almost without exception they invade flesh and other tissues of the body of the living animal. They may block

---

[2] Italic numbers in parentheses refer to Literature Cited.

important ducts and passages and thus impair their functions, and they predispose the animal to various diseases. Even the parasites that ordinarily occur in small numbers may under certain conditions become numerous and as a result of such heavy infection sap the strength and vitality of the host animal.

Two methods of combating parasites are open to the swine raiser. One is to administer drugs to expel the parasites from the bodies of the invaded animals. The other is to outwit and outmaneuver these destroyers of health by protecting the animals from invasion–in other words, to raise the pigs under such conditions that they will not become infected.

The administration of drugs has some inherent disadvantages, one of which is that at least one very important parasite occurs in locations in the body where it is beyond the reach of drugs. Another wanders extensively in the tissues of the body and cannot be expelled until it has settled and become mature, by which time it may have undermined the health of the host.

Prevention of infection by measures designed to break the life cycle of the parasite at its weakest point, the stage on the ground, is in the long run the cheapest method of combating the menace. Such a plan involves raising the animals in clean quarters and on clean temporary pastures away from permanent hog lots and permanent pastures, which are hotbeds of infection. It may be accepted as a fact that the extent of parasitism in swine is proportional to the lack of sanitation. Hogs that are fed on the ground may be heavily infected with parasites, since the animals habitually spend much time on the area where they feed, and most of the droppings, which are the conveyors of parasite infection, are deposited on the feeding lot. The menace of permanent hog pastures has been summarized in the slogan "Permanent pastures perpetuate parasites."

The management practices described in the latter part of this article have proved helpful in controlling parasites on farms where they would otherwise constitute a serious problem. The control measures suggested are based on detailed scientific knowledge of the life histories of the parasites. The facts that must be known include the manner in which a parasite propagates, the stage at which it is infective to swine, the ability of the parasite in the infective stage to maintain itself on pastures and hog lots, the conditions under which pigs become infected, the behaviour of the parasite in the body of the animal, and the damage it inflicts. Unless a farmer has a knowledge of these facts he can do little to overcome such pests.

Essential features of the life cycles of the most important parasites of swine are given in the discussion that follows.

Worm Parasites

Tapeworms

The Pork Bladder Worm

Tapeworms occur in swine only in the larval stage, in which they are known as bladder worms because they are bladder-shaped. Bladder worms are located primarily in the muscles, but they may also invade other tissues of the body.

An important tapeworm of domestic swine in this country is the pork bladder worm (*Cysticercus cellulosae*), a form of the parasite which occurs in the muscles and produces a condition known as measly pork. The muscles chiefly invaded are those of the heart, head, diaphragm, abdomen, and tongue and those used for chewing. The parasite may also occur in the brain and other nerve tissue.

This pork bladder worm is the larval stage of an important tapeworm of man. Pigs become infected by swallowing the eggs or segments containing eggs that have been passed in the feces of infected human beings. In the intestine of the pig, the tiny embryos contained in the tapeworm eggs break the shells and by means of six tiny hooks with which they are equipped bore into the wall of the intestine, where they penetrate the blood vessels. The blood stream carries them throughout the body. When the hatched embryos known as larvae, reach the finest blood vessels (capillaries) they force their way through the blood-vessel wall and burrow into the muscles, where they grow rapidly and develop into bladder worms. They appear as glistening white spots in the muscles, each spot being somewhat larger than a grain of tapioca.

In recent years clinical symptoms of tapeworm infection have seldom been observed in pigs, probably because most infections are very light. In severe infections sensitiveness in the snout and paralysis of the tongue, which may seriously interfere with feeding, have been reported. A slight tap on the end of the nose that would not affect a normal pig may cause an infected animal to squeal with pain. Eventually the animal may become unable to eat and may die of starvation. Blindness may sometimes result from the presence of bladder worms in the brain or in the eyes. Feebleness, shortness of breath, diarrhoea, prostration, and death have been reported as results of a heavy infection.

Bladder worm infection of swine can be diagnosed with certainty as a rule only after the death of the animal, when the parasites may be seen on the surface of the heart and other muscles. In certain countries where the parasite is prevalent and infections are probably severe, inspection of the tongues of live pigs for bladder worms is frequently practiced.

Fortunately, of late years, only a small proportion of hogs in the United States have been infected with the pork bladder worm (pork measles). For example, only 44 cases of infection of swine with bladder worms occurred in Texas during the period 1902 to 1924 (9). From 1930 to 1939, inclusive, only 1 hog out of each 6,000,000 slaughtered under Government supervision was condemned because of infection with this parasite.

The Hydatid

A bladder worm that sometimes occurs in hogs in certain parts of the United States is the hydatid (*Echinococcus granulosus*), the larval stage of an extremely small tapeworm of dogs and wolves. Unlike the parasite that causes pork measles, these bladder worms do not become localized in muscles but are found primarily in the liver and other organs. They vary greatly in size, in many cases being as large as a walnut or larger.

Swine become infected by swallowing the eggs passed in the feces of dogs or wolves harbouring the adult tapeworms. The course of infection is then much the same as that followed by pork bladder worms. No specific symptoms have been associated with the presence of these cysts in swine. Owing to their large size and the fact that they displace normal tissue, however, they may be considered as injurious, particularly when located in the liver. They make the affected tissue unfit for use as food.

Human beings also may become infected with hydatids by swallowing the tapeworm eggs. When swine are slaughtered on the farm, any parts containing these bladder worms should be destroyed and not fed to dogs, since the tapeworm-infected dogs would serve as a reservoir for the infection of additional hogs and possibly of human beings.

The Thin-Necked Bladder Worm

A bladder worm that occasionally parasitizes hogs is the larval stage of another tapeworm of dogs known as the thin-necked bladder worm (technically *Taenia hydatigena*). This large bladder worm sometimes occurs embedded in the liver, but more often it is attached to the abdominal organs or free in the abdominal cavity. It is usually about an inch in diameter but may attain larger sizes. Hogs may acquire infection as a result of swallowing eggs in the droppings of infected dogs.

Light infections probably produce little injury, but it has been stated that heavy infections may be fatal to young pigs, since considerable damage is done to the liver by the migrating larvae. No method is known by which the infection can be diagnosed during the life of the animal.

Flukes

Two species of flukes occur in swine in this country–the lung fluke, *Paragonimus westermanii,* which also occurs in dogs, cats, sheep, and cattle, and occasionally in human beings in other countries, and the liver fluke, *Fasciola hepatica,* which occurs chiefly in cattle and sheep but occasionally in swine. Liver flukes have a complex life history which involves a snail as intermediate host. Hogs become infected as a result of swallowing green forage or water harbouring the metacercariae (flukes in the infective stage) which have emerged from the bodies of snails. Flukes in the adult stages may be found in the bile ducts of the liver. Owing to their relatively infrequent occurrence, liver flukes do not ordinarily constitute a serious problem in swine raising.

Roundworms

Roundworms are the most widespread and undoubtedly the most injurious of the worm parasites that invade the bodies of swine. Almost all organs and tissues of an animal's body may be penetrated by one or more species of roundworms either in their adult or larval (immature) stages. The larvae of some species wander extensively throughout the body of the host and in spite of their small size cause considerable damage to the tissues they invade.

Although a large number of species of roundworms have been reported from swine in the United States, only about 20 species are common. Of these, fortunately, only a few, comparatively are of major importance under ordinary conditions. The swine raiser should nevertheless remember that even species commonly considered to be of little importance damage the tissues in which they are located and are therefore potentially injurious to the health of the animal. Under any of the various conditions that impair the health of growing pigs, such as inadequate nutrition, severe climatic conditions, and disease, parasites that ordinarily occur in small numbers may become a serious problem.

The roundworms considered to be of least importance under ordinary conditions will be discussed briefly. The more important forms will be treated in some detail as a prelude to a discussion of control measures.

Gullet Worms

The gullet worm (technically *Gongylonema pulchrum*) occurs in the lining of the esophagus, or gullet, and in the tongue. In these locations it appears as a white wavy line just beneath the surface. The female worm is about an inch in length and the male somewhat smaller.

Gullet worms are reported to be prevalent in swine in the Middle Atlantic, the Middle Western, and the Pacific Coast States. In a series of post mortem examinations in which the parasites were looked for, gullet worms were found in the esophagi of 14 percent of the swine examined.

Gullet worms have an indirect life history–that is, their development requires that they live for a time in an intermediate host. Eggs of microscopic size, each containing a tiny embryo, are liberated by the female worm into the mouth or esophagus of the infected pig. The eggs are swallowed and pass through the stomach into the small intestine, where they become mixed in the intestinal contents and are voided in the droppings. Various species of dung beetles and certain cockroaches have been reported as capable of serving as intermediate hosts. The insects swallow the eggs while feeding on feces. In the intestine of an insect the tiny embryos break out of the eggs, bore through the intestinal wall, and get into the body cavity, where in about a month they have developed to a stage infective to swine.

Pigs become infected with gullet worms by swallowing the infected beetles. In the body of the pig the young worms are liberated from the insects and make their way to the esophagus and tongue, which they penetrate and in which they grow to maturity.

So far as is known, there are no symptoms that can be definitely ascribed to infections with gullet worms, and in light infections the effect on the host may be slight.

Gullet worms are of importance from the standpoint of human health. A number of cases of infection of human beings have been reported, and infected hogs may serve as reservoirs of such infection.

Stomach Worms

Three species of worms occur in the stomachs of swine in the United States. Two (*Ascarops strongylina* and *Physocephalus sexalatus*) are known as thick stomach worms. The worms of these species are more or less similar in general appearance, being reddish in colour and nearly an inch long in the adult stage. The other species, *Hyostrongylus rubidus* known as the red stomach worm, is a small, delicate, slender, reddish worm about one-fifth inch in length. Owing to its small size and reddish colour, it is difficult to see against the lining of the stomach and may be overlooked by the untrained observer.

Thick stomach worms have an indirect life history and utilize as intermediate hosts a large number of the various species of beetles that feed on dung. The eggs are microscopic in size, practically colourless, and thin-shelled. At the time it is deposited by the female worm each egg contains a tiny embryo. The eggs become mixed with the intestinal contents and pass to the outside with the droppings. Insects feeding on the droppings swallow the eggs, they hatch, and the tiny larvae bore through the intestine into the body cavity of the insect, where during the course of about a month they develop to a stage infective to swine. Hogs feeding on contaminated ground swallow the beetles. In the stomach of the hog the parasites are freed from the bodies of the beetles by the action of the digestive juices. The young worms make their way into the mucous membrane of the stomach, where they grow to maturity.

When stomach worms are present in small numbers the effect on the host animal may not be very great. Symptoms that have been attributed to the parasites in heavy infections are loss of appetite, restlessness, and a great craving for water. Even when the worms are present in small numbers there is generally a thick mucuslike covering on the stomach wall in which the adult worms are buried. Such a condition may well interfere with digestion and contribute to the general unthriftiness common in parasite-infected swine.

Noticeable injuries sometimes result from penetration of the worms into the wall of the stomach. The worms sometimes penetrate deeply, the hole made being similar in appearance to a pinprick. Such lesions may pave the way for bacterial invasion of the stomach wall.

The occurrence of thick stomach worms is widespread in hogs in the United States. In certain of the Midwestern States as many as 90 percent of the animals examined have been found to harbour the worms, and in the Southeastern States, 50 to 80 percent.

One of the thick stomach worms (*Physocephalus sexalatus*) has the peculiar ability to encyst, or form a protective outer covering, and remain alive in the stomach wall of various animals and birds that are not its normal hosts. When the infected insect is swallowed by such a strange host, the young worms make their way into the stomach wall and there surround themselves by a heavy cyst wall, inside of which they remain dormant. When fed to susceptible pigs, such encysted forms were able to develop into mature worms (4). Hence, when steps are taken to control this parasite, consideration must be given to the possibility of its transmission through the medium of snakes, birds, and other small animals that may have become infected and may in turn be eaten by hogs.

Red stomach worms are apparently less common than thick stomach worms. In one section of the United States where the prevalence of these worms has been investigated, as many as 15 to 35 percent of the hogs examined have been found to harbour them.

The life history of the red stomach worm differs from that of the thick stomach worms in that no intermediate host is necessary, the infections being directly acquired. Female worms on the stomach wall produce thin-shelled, partly developed eggs that pass through the intestine of the host and out with its droppings. Development of the eggs then progresses rapidly under favourable conditions of moisture and temperature, and in about 24 to 48 hours a tiny motile embryo has fully formed within the egg. The egg then hatches and the microscopic larva grows and develops, and reaches a stage infective to swine in about 6 days. During this period of growth the larva undergoes one complete and one partial molt. In other words, it completely sheds the outer covering of the body once, and the second time the outer covering becomes loosened and considerably stretched, and a new covering forms underneath. The old unshed covering serves to protect the larva against drying and other injurious environmental conditions. The larva at this stage is said to be ensheathed and is infective to swine.

The infective larvae live in the feces and on the soil beneath and immediately surrounding the fecal mass. Those that are protected from sunlight and drying live for several weeks or months; as more and more eggs are deposited, the soil eventually teems with larvae.

Hogs become infected by swallowing the infective larvae while feeding around droppings. Upon reaching the stomach of the pig, the young worms begin to grow and in the course of about 20 to 25 days reach maturity. The worms then mate, and the females begin to produce eggs.

The damage produced by red stomach worms is sometimes severe. As shown by a number of investigators, erosion (slow destruction) and ulceration of the mucous membrane of the stomach may occur, with extensive formation of mucus. Symptoms that have been associated with infections include diarrhoea, variable appetite, and emaciation; occasionally the animal dies. On the other hand, some investigators consider that the parasite is not particularly harmful unless it is present in association with other disease processes or invades animals whose vitality is depleted, such as young nursing sows or animals fed a deficient diet. Pigs fed an adequate diet and kept under sanitary conditions were not seriously affected by moderate experimental infections, and the worms persisted 6 to 8 months in the absence of reinfections.

Intestinal Threadworms

Adult intestinal threadworms (*Strongyloides ransomi*) are among the smallest of the roundworms that infect swine.

These worm parasites are peculiar in that no males have been found in association with females in the intestine of the swine host. Moreover, in the stages outside the body of the host they may undergo a complex and unusual course of development on soil. The adult female worms are about one-sixth of an inch or less in length. They are whitish and occur embedded more or less deeply in the intestinal tissue, where they may be overlooked even by trained observers.

Intestinal threadworms occur in hogs everywhere. In a series of examinations of swine of all ages, 26 percent were found to harbour these worms. In view of the fact that older animals may develop a resistance to infection, the incidence of the infection in pigs is probably much higher than indicated, since many adult swine were included in the examinations in question. The prevalence of these worms in pigs is illustrated by the fact that they have been found wherever they have been looked for.

Eggs produced by the female threadworms in the intestine of the host usually contain an embryo by the time they reach the exterior. In the feces the microscopic eggs complete their development and hatch within a few hours. The larvae follow one of two courses of development. Some larvae develop within a few days, during which they have undergone one complete and one incomplete molt, to a stage in which they are infective to swine. Others develop into male and female worms, so small as to be almost microscopic, which are not infective to swine. In the latter case the worms mate, and the female produces numerous eggs, from which tiny larvae hatch and soon develop to the infective stage. This dual method of development serves to increase greatly the number of infective larvae on the ground, and hence the probability that pigs will become severely infected is increased.

A pig may become infected by swallowing the infective larvae, or the larvae may penetrate its skin when the animal is rooting or lying on the ground. In either case the larvae get into the blood stream and are carried to the lungs. Here they break out of the tiny blood vessels, get into the air spaces (bronchioles), and crawl up the air passages into the throat, where they are swallowed. During this journey the larvae increase greatly in size. After being swallowed they pass down the esophagus and through the stomach and ultimately reach the small intestine. They attain maturity in about 7 days after entering the body of the animal.

Threadworms in small numbers may have little noticeable effect on pigs fed adequate amounts of a well-balanced diet, even though the infection may persist throughout the life of the animal. The number of threadworm eggs passed in the feces of adult animals that have developed a resistance to infection is usually very small. When the vitality of the animal becomes depleted, however–as in nursing sows, for example–the worms may gain the upper hand and produce vast numbers of eggs. This favours infection of the young pigs. In massive infecitons pigs may suffer from severe diarrhoea. As a result of penetration o the larvae, pigs may also develop a skin eruption, which is usually more severe in young than in older animals. Little is known concerning the number of worms necessary to produce noticeable symptoms in pigs, but it has been estimated that infected pigs that were emaciated and suffering from severe diarrhoea harbored 10,000 to 25,000 threadworms in the intestine.

The infective larvae of threadworms are capable of penetrating the unbroken skin of human beings. It has been observed that when large numbers of larvae penetrate at one time, severe itching occurs, followed later by a marked puffiness, which may persist several days, at the site of penetration. Persons walking barefoot over ground infested with infective larvae of threadworms may develop a swelling of the feet as a result of penetration of the larvae. So far as is known, threadworms of swine do not grow to maturity in man.

Nodular Worms

Nodular worms are parasites of the blind gut (cecum) and large intestine and derive their common name from the fact that they produce nodules, or lumps, of varying sizes in the wall of the large intestine and cecum. Nodular worms are perhaps the commonest of the worm parasites of swine. In the southeastern part of the United States, practically all hogs raised under ordinary condition may be infected.

Nodular worms are slender, whitish to grayish in colour, and one-third to one-half inch in length. Four species occur in swine. One (*Oesophagostomum dentatum*) is found in practically all parts of the United States and in southern Canada. The three other species, *O. longicaudum* (the long-tailed nodular worm), *O. brevicaudum* (the short-tailed nodular worm), and *O. georgianum* are found chiefly in the southern part of the United States. The last-named species is found only occasionally. Nodular worms differ from some of the other worm parasites in that they may infect older animals as heavily as younger animals, or even more heavily. An infected animal may harbour several thousand worms.

The various species of nodular worms differ considerably in their effect on the host animal. *Oesophagostomum dentatum* and *O. brevicaudum*, the short-tailed forms, are apparently the least injurious from the standpoint of gross damage to the intestine. The nodules caused by these forms ordinarily are not much larger than the head of a pin and are only moderately inflamed. *O. longicaudum* may produce large nodules that often become secondarily infected with bacteria.

The life histories of all the species of nodular worms are in general quite similar. Since the course of development of the long-tailed form has been worked out in more or less detail, it is used here as an example:

The adult worms of *Oesophagostomum longicaudum* are localized in the cecum and large intestine of the host animal. The females deposit large numbers of partly developed, thin-shelled eggs, which become mixed with the intestinal contents and are eventually eliminated with the droppings. Under favourable conditions of moisture and temperature these eggs develop rapidly in the feces and in about 24 to 48 hours a larva of microscopic size emerges from each. The larvae live in or beneath the pile of fecal material and on the surrounding soil, if it is moist and shaded. After about 3 to 5 days of further development they become infective to swine. The infective larvae are very numerous; in a small lump of feces or a small handful of soil there may be thousands. Infective nodular worm larvae do not like either strong light or complete darkness but prefer a subdued light. If placed in a glass dish containing water half of which is shaded, the larvae will collect at the juncture of the shaded and unshaded portions. When larvae are able to find favourable conditions in nature, as at the base of grass on pastures, they may survive 14 months or longer. They are unable to withstand complete drying longer than a few hours. When the surface of the soil dries, they may migrate downward to the layer of moist soil underneath. When the surface of the soil becomes moist again, they may return upward where the chances of coming in contact with host animals are greater. The larvae also migrate short distances up the stems and blades of grass or other objects wet with dew or ram, and this increases their chances of being swallowed by hogs grazing on the moist grass. Also when feces containing the eggs are buried, as by plowing, the eggs will hatch and the larvae will migrate upward. In plowed fields where the surface of the soil becomes thoroughly dried, however, many of the larvae are apparently unable to reach the surface.

Observations on farms have shown that pigs become infected with nodular worms as a result of swallowing the larvae while feeding on contaminated ground or grazing on contaminated pastures. After being swallowed, the larvae pass through the stomach into the small intestine and thence into the large intestine. By this time the protective sheath has been discarded, and the larvae penetrate into the wall of the large intestine and the blind gut. Despite their small size, frequently they severely injure the tissue immediately surrounding them as they bore into the wall. Often this causes an intense inflammation, and in 48 hours or sooner a small nodule, or elevation, has been formed at the place where the larva penetrated.

Inside the cyst the young worm grows and develops for about 2 to 3 weeks. During this time it increases greatly in size, and the cyst also enlarges. The young worm reaches a stage in which it very closely resembles the adult worm except that it is smaller. It then breaks out of the cyst and moves into the lumen, or cavity, of the intestine, where it continues its development. About 5 to 7 weeks after the infection the worms are fully grown, have mated and begun to produce eggs, and the cycle begins all over again.

The precise effect of nodular worms on pigs has not been definitely ascertained. Most of the information available comes from observations of clinical cases of nodular worm infection. It has been stated that development of the nodules in the intestine may interfere with the proper absorption of food material and consequently affect the health of the host animal. There is also danger of infection of the nodules by bacteria; it is the observation of the writer that marked secondary infection of nodules is common in infections with the long-tailed nodular worm. According to some investigators, there is clinical evidence to suggest that in addition to the irritation produced by the nodules, a toxic substance produced by the worms is absorbed into the system of the host and results in a mild toxemia.

In nodules containing young *Oesophagostomum longicaudum*, a fluid surrounds the worm inside the cyst. As the worm grows, the cyst enlarges greatly, and the amount of fluid increases. Shortly before the worm is ready to move into the lumen of the intestine the cyst wall ruptures and the fluid surrounding the worm escapes and may be absorbed into the system of the animal. Although the amount of fluid in one cyst is probably negligible, the amount from thousands of cysts would be considerable. When large numbers of cysts rupture at about the same time, the animal may well suffer from toxemia if this fluid is absorbed. In this connection it has been possible to detect in the muscle tissue of infected swine the presence of substances similar to those composing the bodies of nodular worms. Although the source of these substances is not definitely known, they may have come in part from the cysts.

The adult worms may also damage the intestine by producing irritation and inflammation, according to some investigators. Weakness, anemia, emaciation, diarrhoea, and general unthriftiness have been reported to be common results of infection with these parasites.

An important economic result of nodular worm infection of swine is the unsuitability of the severely infected intestines for use either as sausage casings or as food. In certain parts of the country the large intestines of pigs (chitterlings) constitute a more or less common article of diet. Since the parasites are not known to be transmissible to man, chitterlings showing small numbers of pinhead-sized nodules without inflammation, such as result from infection with *Oesophagostomum dentatum*, are safe for human consumption after the lesions are trimmed out, but inflammation and secondary infection, such as often occur in infections with the long-tailed nodular worm, make the intestine unfit for use as food. Intestines studded with nodules are generally weak and tear easily, and this largely destroys their value for use as sausage casings. It may be considered, then, that nodular worm infections cause considerable losses to the meat industry, which are passed on to the farmer in the form of lower market prices.

Whipworms

Whipworms (*Trichuris suis*) inhabit the blind gut and large intestine of swine. Little is known concerning the prevalence of this parasite except in the Southeastern States, where 23 percent of all the swine examined were found to harbour this parasite, the number of worms ranging from 2 to 163 per animal.

The whipworm is about 1 to 2 inches in length. The body is composed of a long slender part resembling the lash of a whip and a shorter thick part resembling the whip stock; hence the name "whipworm." The slender part of the worm bears the mouth at the tip and is about twice as long as the thick part. The male is slightly smaller than the female, and the end of the thick part of the male is sharply coiled. Whipworms attach themselves to the intestine by sewing the long whiplike part of the body into the tissues.

The eggs deposited by adult female whipworms are keg-shaped and have brownish-coloured, thick shells. They are produced in large numbers, become mixed with the intestinal contents of the host, and are then eliminated with the feces. The eggs are undeveloped when passed. They develop in the feces, a tiny embryo forming within each egg, but they do not hatch there; they remain quiescent until they are swallowed by a host animal or until they die. Eggs of whipworms develop slowly. In some cases the development of the larvae requires several months, but under certain conditions of high humidity and temperature, it may be accomplished in about a month.

Pigs become infected with whipworms by swallowing the infective eggs when feeding on soil where they are present. The eggs hatch in the stomach and intestine, and the larvae make their way to the blind gut, where they grow to maturity in about 10 weeks or longer.

Well-fed pigs harbouring small numbers of whipworms usually show no recognizable symptoms, and the infection is generally short-lived, lasting only a few weeks. In massive infections growth may be noticeably retarded. The writer has observed heavily infected pigs whose strength appeared to ebb slowly until they finally died. Upon examination, the blind gut of such animals was found to be inflamed, greatly thickened, and festooned with whipworms.

Very little information is available as to how long whipworm eggs will remain alive on soil. It is known, however, that eggs of the whipworm that parasitizes human beings and those of the whipworm of dogs are killed rather quickly by drying and do not live long on soil where shade is lacking and moisture is not abundant. The same is probably true of the eggs of the swine whipworm, since it was observed at the Beltsville Research Center, Beltsville, Md., in the summer of 1940, that whipworm eggs on a hog lot lost their vitality about 2 months after the area was cleared of trees and other vegetation.

The species of whipworm found in human beings is closely related to that found in swine, and for a time the two were thought to be identical. Under certain conditions it was believed human beings might become infected with whipworms as a result of swallowing eggs that had passed out of swine. Recently, however, study of the two forms has confirmed the conclusions of the scientist who originally described the parasite many years ago that the species are separate and distinct. There is, therefore, little likelihood of infection of man with the swine whipworm.

Lungworms

Lungworms are known to be among the most widespread of the parasites that infect swine. Reports indicate that this parasite may be found in swine in all parts of the United States and in Canada. In the southeastern section of the United States 70 percent or more of the swine examined were found to be infected. Lungworms do great damage to young pigs. It is believed by some investigators that they sap the strength of the animal, ruin its appetite, and make it short-winded. There is also evidence to indicate that these parasites may be instrumental in the spread of swine influenza, a very important virus disease (*17*).

Lungworms are whitish, threadlike roundworms that may attain a length of about 2 inches. They commonly occur in the smaller air passages of the lungs (bronchioles) and may be found by cutting off the tips of the lobes of the lungs and squeezing the tissues, which forces the worms out of the bronchioles. In heavy infections the worms may also be found in the larger air passages (trachea and bronchi).

Three species of lungworms belonging to two genera are of common occurrence in swine in this country. The two most common forms, *Metastrongylus elongatus* and *Choerostrongylus pudendotectus*, are usually present in about equal numbers and are of widespread occurrence. The third species, *Metastrongylus salmi*, is found chiefly in swine raised in the South; generally only a small percentage of hogs harbour this form, and the infections are usually very light.

Recently it was found that the life history is indirect and involves as intermediate hosts various species of earthworms, particularly redstriped worms of the genus *Helodrilus*, which are found chiefly in manure piles and rich, fecest-contaminated soil. The common garden or orchard earthworm (*Lumbricus*) may also serve as intermediate host.

Female lungworms produce large numbers of thick-shelled eggs each containing a tiny embryo. The eggs are coughed up, swallowed, and eliminated in the feces of the host. Earthworms feeding on the feces swallow the eggs, which hatch in the earthworm's intestine. The tiny lungworm larvae bore into the glandular portion of the intestine (the portion that contains the calciferous glands) and also get into one or all of the five to seven pairs of hearts of the earthworm. In about 3 weeks to a month the lungworm larvae have completed their development and are capable of producing an infection in a pig that swallows the earthworm.

In the body of the pig the lungworm larvae, liberated from the earthworm by the digestive juices, migrate by way of the lymphatic and blood-circulatory systems to the lungs, where they become localized, complete development, and begin to produce eggs in about 1½ months.

Lungworm eggs are long-lived. On soil under favourable conditions of moisture and shade they probably survive for years. Earthworms infected with lungworm larvae have been found in a hog lot abandoned for approximately 4 years. During this time the lot apparently had remained grown up to weeds and the soil had remained moist. Earthworms kept in samples of this soil became infected with lungworms, showing that lungworm eggs were present (22). In contrast to this, eggs on dry soil at Beltsville, Md., failed to survive more than 1 month during the summer. The eggs are very resistant to low temperatures when adequate moisture is present and have been found to survive continuous freezing at temperatures of 14° to 20° F. for more than a year. Eggs buried in soil survived for periods of several months where grass or other vegetation was growing and the roots penetrated to the level of the eggs. Where the soil was bare of vegetation the period of survival was much shorter (7). Such observations show that areas extensively contaminated with feces of lungworm-infected swine may remain dangerous to susceptible swine for a number of years unless the animals can be prevented from eating the earthworm intermediate hosts.

The presence of lungworms and the feeding of there parasites in the bronchioles of the host are considered to be a source of irritation to the animal. The worms also block up the air passages and interfere mechanically with breathing. One of the most outstanding symptoms of lungworm infection is a cough. Even lightly infected animals may be subject to fits of coughing, which weakens the animal and lowers its vitality. Coughing is more pronounced after exertion of any kind.

The irritation to the lungs arising from the presence of the worms and their feeding, together with the plugging of the bronchioles, results in a consolidation, or hardening, of the lung tissue surrounding the sites occupied by the worms, and hard nodules soon form in the tissue. During the early stages of invasion, hemorrhages may appear on the surface of the lungs. In infections of long standing the tips of the lungs become grayish or whitish and hard.

Animals infected with lungworms frequently tend to go off feed. A change of diet usually remedies this condition for a time, but it may return. Ultimately unthriftiness and failure to grow normally result.

Kidney Worms

The swine kidney worm, technically *Stephanurus dentatus*, causes heavy losses to southern swine raisers and to the meat industry. It is probably one of the most injurious pests with which the producer in the South has to contend and one which he must assiduously combat in order to make swine raising profitable. In the South losses from trimming of infected carcasses and from condemnation of livers, kidneys, and other organs damaged by the parasite have been estimated at approximately 27 cents per animal slaughtered. Since about 10 million hogs raised in the Southern States are slaughtered annually in Government-inspected abattoirs, the annual loss from kidney worms may be estimated at more than 2.7 million dollars. In addition producers suffer losses from arrested growth and development of swine and imperfect utilization of feed, which may result from interference by the parasite with the proper functioning of important organs and tissues.

Although kidney worms are most common in the South, increasing reports of the occurrence of these worms in swine in various parts of the Northern States and even in Canada indicate that the parasite may be spreading northward. If it gains a foothold in breeding swine in the North it may well become a serious problem there.

Kidney worms are thick-bodied black-and-white worms which, when fully grown, may attain a length of 2 inches. Mature worms may be found in the kidneys and in cysts in the ureters (tubes leading from the kidneys to the bladder). In addition to the worms these cysts often contain a greenish or whitish pus. Immature worms invade the liver, kidney fat, blood vessels, lungs, and other locations outside the digestive tract. Wherever they are located, kidney worms destroy vital tissue.

Mature female kidney worms embedded in the kidneys and ureters produce large numbers of dark-coloured, partly developed eggs which they deposit in the cavities of the kidneys and of the ureters through perforations in the walls of these tubes. The eggs pass down the ureters into the bladder, where they collect until discharged with the urine. As many as 700,000 to 1,000,000 eggs have been observed in the urine passed by a moderately infected hog in 1 day. Eggs that fall on moist, shaded soil develop rapidly, and in about 24 to 48 hours, depending on temperature conditions, a tiny larva hatches from each egg. The larva develops rapidly and during the course of 3 to 5 days undergoes one complete and one partial molt, after which it is infective to the host animal.

Observations under actual farm conditions have shown that the larvae are extremely exacting in their requirements for shade and moisture (*16, 19*), as described later.

Swine become infected with kidney worms as a result of swallowing the infective larvae while feeding or rooting in contaminated soil. French scientists first observed that kidney worm larvae may penetrate the skin of pigs. Later this was confirmed by Australian scientists. In the United States, however, it was found that larvae placed on the unbroken skin of pigs were unable to penetrate it. It was finally ascertained that they are able to penetrate the unbroken skin of pigs, provided some object is available against which they can brace themselves in order to force their way in (*20*). Particles of soil or mud sticking to the bodies of swine might provide the necessary condition.

It has been thought that swine may become infected as a result of frequenting wallows contaminated with the urine of animals infected with kidney worms. Careful studies have failed to disclose the presence of larvae in these locations, however.

Having once entered the bodies of swine, kidney worm larvae get into the blood stream and are carried to the liver, lungs, and other organs. Those that arrive in the liver and large blood vessels adjacent to that organ grow and develop to many times their original size over a period that may last 4 or 5 months. During this time the worms in the liver burrow extensively through the tissue, particularly just beneath the capsule (membranous covering), where they leave crooked, bloody tracks. Many of the parasites remain in this organ until they die and degenerate (*14*). Others break out through the liver capsule and migrate among the abdominal organs until they reach the kidney region, where some immediately penetrate the kidneys and ureters and others come to rest in the fat surrounding the kidneys, causing considerable inflammation there.

The time required for the worms to reach maturity in different swine hosts varies considerably. According to some investigators, the worms that become established in the walls of the ureters and in the tissue of the kidney proper begin to produce eggs about 6 or 7 months after first entering the body of the animal. On the other hand, the worms were found to be still immature in a pig slaughtered 12 months after being experimentally infected.

So far as is known there are no readily observable symptoms peculiar to kidney worm infection. Infected animals frequently discharge pus in the urine, particularly when the infection is heavy. However, this has not been found to be a reliable criterion of infection, as it naturally would not occur until the worms had reached the kidneys and set up disorders in those organs, which as previously pointed out might take 6 months or longer. It has been shown that the growth rate of 2- or 3-week-old pigs is markedly retarded following infection (*14*). Posterior paralysis (paralysis of the hindquarters) may sometimes occur as a result of injury to the spinal cord by migrating kidney worms.

The principal injury inflicted by kidney worms occurs in the liver. If the lesions caused by the migrations of the worms have healed, the liver at autopsy appears badly scarred, showing hard grayish areas, which are sometimes small, circumscribed, and more or less shallow and sometimes large and deep. Completely healed lesions often do not contain worms. Incompletely healed and unhealed lesions are usually soft and may contain pus and live worms or dead worms that may be partly disintegrated. In addition, the infected livers are often covered with a fibrinous deposit which sometimes causes them to adhere to adjacent tissue. Similar lesions are often found in lungs and other organs.

Liver destruction retards the growth and impairs the health of the infected animal. According to some observers, death commonly occurs among young pigs as a result of the extensive destruction of the liver tissue and the effects of the marked changes accompanying such destruction (*3*).

As previously mentioned, kidney worms inflict extensive damage on the kidneys and ureters. An important and quite common accompaniment of kidney worm infection is a condition known as hydronephrosis, which was first noted in 1923 by an Australian scientist. This is the result of the destruction of kidney tissue until a portion of it is replaced by a watery cyst. The condition is undoubtedly harmful to the animal, since it hampers the functioning of the kidney. In addition, the presence in the walls of the ureters of cystic cavities containing worms often has the effect of thickening the walls to such an extent that the passage is almost stopped up (Fig. 2). The writer has often seen ureters with walls so inflamed and thickened as a result of invasion by kidney worms that a darning needle would

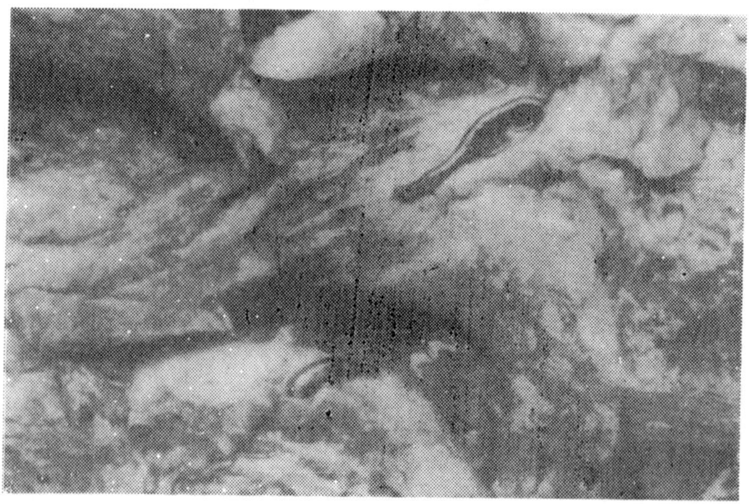

Fig. 2: Portion of the ureter of a hog infected with kidney worms, two of which are visible.

scarcely pass through the opening. Such a condition probably results in the retention of a certain amount of urine, which would interfere with the proper functioning of the kidney and therefore impair the health of the animal.

More or less extensive thickening and inflammation of the urinary bladder has been observed by the writer to be common in swine infected with kidney worm. The daily accumulation of eggs in the bladder irritates its delicate tissues. Furthermore, worms frequently become dislodged from their locations in the kidneys and ureters and pass down to the bladder, where they generally rupture and become partly disintegrated, releasing the contents of their bodies, which may also serve to irritate the bladder.

According to Australian investigators, the effect of kidney worms on the general health and condition of an animal may be so great that it becomes possible to pick out the carcasses of infected pigs in abattoirs by their appearance, which is less pleasing and leaner than that of the carcasses of normal pigs. This poor condition is the direct result of unthriftiness and slow growth resulting from various injuries caused by the worms.

Figure 3 illustrates the effect of kidney worms and other parasites on the growth of pigs. The two carcasses shown are of animals the same age; the smaller animal probably became infected with kidney worms early in life, while the larger was raised free of parasites. Retardation of growth caused by kidney worms is a costly matter to the swine raiser even if considered only from the standpoint of market value. It is evident that the smaller animal the carcass of which is pictured here could be expected to sell for only a small fraction of what the larger animal would bring. Furthermore, during its lifetime it probably consumed as much feed as the larger pig, and perhaps more.

The presence in the liver of worms or lesions makes the invaded tissue unsuitable for food. In light infections, where only a small number of superficial lesions occur in livers, the affected portions can be trimmed out, but even this reduces the market value of the organ. Loin muscles are frequently invaded by kidney worms, necessitating considerable trimming of these valuable parts of carcasses. Occasionally kidney worms migrate to other parts of the muscle structure. The writer has frequently observed lesions in hams made by kidney worms burrowing through the flesh; such meat is

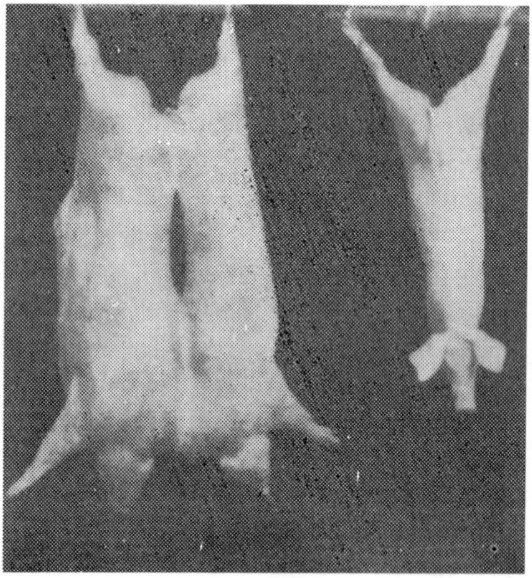

Fig. 3: Carcasses of two pigs the same age. The smaller was infected with kidney worms and other parasites, while the larger had been protected from these pests.

unfit for food. Another loss is the spoilage of kidney fat, the so-called leaf fat. Many kidney worms come to rest in the fat surrounding the kidneys, where they irritate the tissues and are soon surrounded by areas of inflammation which make the fat inedible. The pancreas, spleen, lungs, and other organs are also frequently invaded by the worms, and these parts become unfit for use as food.

All such losses are ultimately borne by the farmer in the form of lowered market prices. In some areas where kidney worms and other parasites are prevalent, a blanket reduction in price is made to compensate for losses due to parasites and other diseases and conditions. In the last analysis, therefore, the producer of hogs infected with kidney worms is the principal loser.

In areas where kidney worms are prevalent and hogs and cattle occupy the same pastures, cattle also sometimes become infected.

Hookworms

Several species of hookworms have been reported as being found in the small intestines of swine the world over. Only one species, technically called *Crassisoma urosubulatum,* however, is common in swine in the United States. It occurs chiefly in the southern part of the country and is a white, fat-bodied worm that may reach a length of about one-fourth of an inch. About 11 percent of the swine examined for this parasite have been found infected. The life history of this hookworm has not been demonstrated in its entirety, although it is probably similar to that of other hookworms. The thin-shelled, partly developed eggs become mixed in the intestinal contents of the host and pass out with the droppings. On soil the eggs complete development and hatch within a few days. The larvae undergo one complete and one incomplete molt, after which they are infective to swine. It is not known how long the larvae will live on soil or how they are affected by sunlight, drying, and other climatic conditions. Infection probably results from swallowing the larvae along with feed and water, although they may also penetrate the skin, as do the larvae of other hookworms.

This hookworm parasite of swine was first seen by an Italian scientist in 1909. He noted that the worms attach themselves to the intestine by sucking a portion of the tissue into their mouths. Since the mouths of the worms are provided with sharp cutting plates, or teeth, they may lacerate the tissues and cause bleeding. It was noted that the worms caused punctiform hemorrhages, and that the presence of the parasites was associated with a catarrhal condition of the intestine.

Since the worms apparently lacerate the tissues and cause hemorrhages, they probably suck blood. When present in large numbers, therefore, they may cause anemia, just as do the hookworms parasitic in other animals. In light infections the worms probably do little noticeable injury. It has been observed that a residuum of infection is sometimes present in the breeding stock on farms and that under certain conditions that are not well understood the pigs become heavily infected. In such cases the worms probably contribute to the general unthriftiness common in parasite-infected animals.

Thorn-Headed Worms

Zoologically, the thorn-headed worms (technically called *Macrocanthorhynchus hirudinaceus*) which occur in the large intestine of swine are not true roundworms. These parasites, known as acanthocephalids, are considered by some investigators to be related to both the roundworms and the tapeworms. Unlike the roundworms but like the tapeworms, they have no intestine, and a spiny protuberance at one end serves to attach the worm to the intestine of the host. Like the roundworms, however, they are cylindrical, elongate, and gradually tapering toward the hind end, and the sexes are separate. The female worms may reach an extreme length of 12 or more inches, while the males, which have a small swelling at the end of the tail, are somewhat shorter.

These worms attach themselves to the wall of the small intestine by means of a spiny proboscis, or snout. They may not remain attached to anyone spot, however, but may migrate from place to place in the small intestine. At the site of attachment a nodule, or swelling, forms as the result of injury to the tissues by the spiny proboscis; there are usually more nodules than worms present. Fresh nodules are generally inflamed, while older ones may be either hard or secondarily infected with bacteria.

Adult female thorn-headed worms produce numerous thick-shelled, brownish eggs, each containing a fully developed larva. One female may produce as many as 600,000 or more eggs a day at the peak of her egg-producing capacity. The thick shells protect the larvae from drying and from other deleterious environmental conditions. Eggs have been kept in a dried condition for more than a year without apparent effect on the larvae. They are also able to withstand prolonged freezing and may survive temperatures as high as 150° F. The larvae inside the eggs may survive for long periods on soil; eggs on soil at Beltsville, Md., have retained their vitality as long as 4½ years.

Thorn-headed worms have an indirect life cycle. White grubs, the larvae of June bugs (May beetles), rose chafers, and other similar insects may serve as the intermediate hosts. The grubs feeding on manure or on soil contaminated with the feces of infected swine swallow the parasite eggs. The eggs hatch in the intestine of the grub, and within a few hours the tiny larvae penetrate into the wall of the gut. After a period of growth and development lasting about 2 weeks, during which they have greatly increased in size, the parasites migrate into the body cavity of the grub and become sausage-shaped; at this stage they are large enough to be visible to the naked eye.

After further growth and development they reach a stage in which they are infective to swine. At this stage they consist chiefly of a large spiny proboscis invaginated into, or sheathed in a bladderlike appendage so that they somewhat resemble bladder worms.

Development to the infective stage is accomplished in about 7 to 12 weeks, depending on temperature and the stage of development of the host grub; there is evidence that the rate of development of the parasite is speeded up during pupation of the grub. Adult beetles are capable of harbouring the parasite in the infective stage.

Swine rooting in manure piles, strawstacks, or the rich soil of barn-yards or low-lying pastures may find and swallow white grubs, of which they are very fond; they probably also find and eat the beetles during the season when these insects are common. In the body of the hog the infective thorn-headed worm larvae are freed from the body of the insect by the action of the digestive juices. In the small intestine the larvae extend the proboscis and attach themselves to the wall of the intestine, mate, and began to produce eggs in about 3 to 4 months. In the intestine of the hog the worms may grow at the rate of about an inch a mouth. Egg-producing maturity is usually reached before the worms attain their full growth.

The effect of thorn-headed worms on swine is not well understood, although it is known that these worms contribute their share to the general unthriftiness that is commonly associated with parasitic infections. Loss of appetite, constipation, and restlessness have been attributed to infection with these worms, and it has been stated that the parasites often kill young pigs. Occasionally the injury inflicted on the intestine by the proboscis is so deep that the intestinal wall is perforated and the delicate lining of the abdominal cavity becomes inflamed, a condition known as peritonitis. There have been cases in which the entire worm has broken through the intestinal wall and entered the body cavity of the animal. Such a condition may well produce a fatal peritonitis.

An important effect of infection by thorn-headed worms is a marked weakening of the small intestine. In some cases the infected intestines have only about half the strength of uninfected intestines. It has been observed that the intestine is often weakest at a point some distance from the worms. The weakened condition of the intestine makes it unfit for use as sausage casings, and this causes financial loss to the packers which may be passed on to the farmer in the form of lowered market prices.

Large Intestinal Roundworms (Ascarids)

The large intestinal roundworm, or ascarid, parasitic in the small intestine of swine, is probably the most commonly observed and one of the most injurious of all the worm parasites of these animals. It is widespread throughout the world. In the United States, from 20 to 74 percent or more of the hogs examined for this parasite have been found to be infected.

The worm is known as *Ascaris lumbricoides* var. *suis* to distinguish it from *A. lumbricoides*, a worm that occurs in human beings and is presumably closely related to the one in swine, from which it cannot be distinguished by any characteristics of form. Usually reddish or pinkish in colour, the adult worm is about as thick as an ordinary lead pencil and may reach a length of 12 inches or more.

The normal location of the adult worms is in the small intestine, but wandering adults may occur in the stomach, the large intestine, the bile ducts of the liver, or the gall bladder, and they are often seen in the feces of infected animals. The young (larval) worms migrate extensively in the body of the host and during these migrations appear in the blood stream, the liver, the lungs, and other organs and tissues.

At first the life history of this parasite was not well understood. About 1916 an English investigator found that the life cycle is direct. A few years later two American scientists confirmed his work and demonstrated the following points by a series of carefully planned experiments:

(1) Eggs eliminated by female worms in the intestines of pigs are undeveloped. When incubated at a temperature of about 33° C. (91° F.), the eggs may complete development in about 10 days. Longer periods are required at lower temperatures.

(2) The embryonated eggs, if swallowed by a suitable host animal, hatch in the small intestine. The young larvae penetrate the wall of the alimentary tract and, apparently aided by the circulation, migrate to the liver and lungs, being found in the liver as early as 2 days after infection and in the lungs 3 days after infection. Larvae are most numerous in the lungs 10 days after the infection, becoming scarce in

the liver as they become numerous in the lungs. During the period of migration to the liver and lungs, they may also migrate into the spleen, thyroid, pancreas, and other locations in the body.

(3) In the lungs the larvae, which have developed to 5 to 10 times their original size and may be visible to the unaided eye, break out of the capillaries, migrate up the air passages to the throat, are swallowed, and appear in the small intestine as early as 6 days after infection.

(4) In pigs the ascarids develop to maturity within about 2½ months after infection. Some larvae die during their migrations in the body, and those that settle in organs other than the liver and lungs are relatively short-lived.

The course of migration of ascarid larvae in the body of the pig is illustrated in figure 4.

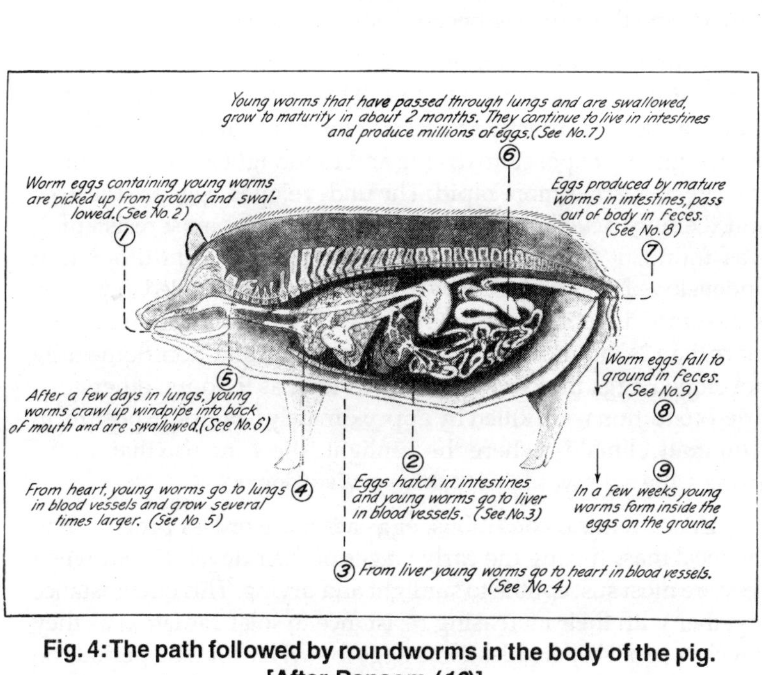

Fig. 4: The path followed by roundworms in the body of the pig. [After Ransom (*12*)].

The eggs of ascarids have a thick, rough shell which makes them resistant to unfavourable environmental conditions. They are therefore able to survive prolonged exposure to freezing temperatures and to drying, and they are killed by few strong chemicals. The eggs are also very long-lived, having been kept alive in the laboratory as long as 5 years. Eggs in cultivated soil have remained alive and been able to infect pigs after approximately 4½ years.

The egg production of adult female ascarids is enormous. It has been estimated that a full-grown female may contain as many as 26 or 27 million eggs, and it has been shown that a single female worm may give off as many as 250,000 eggs a day. This, it can be seen, would result in rapid accumulation of enormous numbers of eggs on the soil where even a few infected hogs are kept. Soil is not necessary for the development of the eggs; they will develop on wood, brick, or concrete floors–in fact, anywhere that slight moisture is present. The eggs are sticky and adhere to the floors and walls of pens, and vigorous cleaning is necessary to dislodge them. When pens are cleaned in the ordinary way, without washing, many eggs remain, and the premises become potential sources of infection.

Although, as pointed out, ascarid eggs are quite resistant to many inimical environment factors, it has been observed that when they are exposed directly to sunlight for a time, many of them die. When eggs are exposed to drying and to sunlight at the same time, the rate of death is more rapid. The undeveloped eggs are the least and the fully developed (embryonated) eggs the most resistant. It was found in tests carried out under tropical conditions that undeveloped eggs protected by a thin layer of water failed to survive exposure to direct sunlight for more than 3 hours, and none survived more than 2¾ hours when exposed in a dried condition. Some fully developed eggs in water survived as long as 9 hours; others in a dried condition were killed by approximately 5 hours' exposure. In temperate climates, where the sunlight is less intense than in the Tropics, the eggs would probably survive longer.

Under natural conditions, eggs are more or less protected by the fecal mass during the early stages of their development when they are most susceptible to sunlight and drying. This circumstance together with their increasing resistance to solar radiation as they develop, probably enables some eggs to survive for long periods on soil even though unprotected by vegetation. Nevertheless sunlight and drying are among the most effective of the measures which the farmer has at his disposal in his war on these parasites.

The damage inflicted by ascarids may be sufficiently great at times to cause the death of heavily infected animals. While the effects produced by moderate and light infections are correspondingly less severe, even these may stunt the animal. An instance in which the rate of growth and general condition of a pig infected with ascarids was compared with that of a pig of the same age kept free from these pests illustrates this point (5). At slightly over 3 months of age the worm-free pig weighed 82 pounds and the infected pig, 10¾ pounds. A large part of the visible damage inflicted by these parasites occurs in the liver and lungs and is produced by the larvae in their migrations through the body of the animal. In heavy infections the damage is so extensive that by the time the worms have appeared in the intestines the health of the animal may have been undermined to such an extent that it may never fully recover. During the migration of the larvae through the lungs, the pig may have difficulty in breathing and may contract pneumonia and die. Infected pigs commonly show symptoms known as thumps–laboured breathing often accompanied by a deep, harsh cough, which is more pronounced after exertion. Although thumps in young pigs may be caused by conditions other than ascarid infection, this is probably the commonest cause in growing pigs kept on permanent pastures. Small hemorrhages and whitish pneumonic areas may also appear in the lungs after extensive invasion by ascarid larvae.

Although the injuries to the liver heal as a general rule they are sometimes so severe as to leave permanent scars which appear at, times as small pearly-white spots. Sometimes these scars are so numerous as to dot the entire surface of the liver. It has been stated that the livers of about 35 percent of the swine slaughtered in some regions show this condition.

The damage produced by the adult worms in the intestine is less spectacular and less definite. Digestive disturbances, capricious appetite, and retarded growth and development have been associated with the presence of adult ascarids in the intestine. In fact, growth may be retarded to such as extent that it is impossible tc get the animals to a marketable weight soon enough to be profitable. The presence of the parasites in the intestine is frequently associated with a reddish slime with a distinctive odour on the wall of the intestine.

A frequent result of ascarid infection of swine is a generalized icterus (yellows). Adult worms occasionally migrate into and plug the bile ducts of the liver, stopping the flow of bile into the intestine. The bile is then distributed by the, blood stream through the body of the animal lodges in the tissues, and gives the flesh a yellowish colour, making it unfit for food. Since such carcasses are rejected and condemned under Federal and equally competent State and local meat-inspection procedures, the animals are almost a total loss.

Protozoan Parasites

The most common of the protozoan parasites belong to four general groups known as amoebae, balantidia, coccidia, and sarcosporidia. The amoebae and the balantidia are of especial importance because they are indistinguishable, for the most part, from similar protozoa that sometimes produce dysentery in man. The coccidia that infect swine are distinct from the coccidia that occur in other animals and in man.

The conditions under which protozoa produce harmful effects in pigs are not well understood. Under ordinary conditions they often appear to do little if any damage. However, the pigs generally become infected with these parasites within a few days after they are born, when the young animal is adjusting itself to life and its resistance is low. Hence the parasites may produce injuries that may not be apparent at once but that may show up later in the form of unthriftiness.

Amoebae

Several species of amoebae, belonging to the genera *Endamoeba, Endolimax*, and *Iodamoeba*, may occur in pigs. The most common are certain species of the *Endamoeba*, three of which are often found in pigs, but considerable difference of opinion exists as to their importance in causing sickness in the young animals. For a number of years investigators have observed these parasites in the intestinal wall of pigs, and some have considered that the organisms act like normal inhabitants of the digestive tract. Others have felt that under certain circumstances the organisms may invade and erode the cells of the intestine, causing dysentery. From time to time outbreaks of dysentery occur in swine that can apparently be attributed to no cause other than amoebae. It has been considered possible also that the pig acts as a reservoir host of the parasite and may be instrumental in bringing about outbreaks of amoebic dysentery in man.

The amoebae may merely live in the cavity of the intestine, or they may invade the tissue cells, where they may well become decidedly harmful. In the intestine the active forms multiply by division of their bodies. Under certain conditions the organism becomes rounded and secretes a heavy cyst wall about itself. Such cysts are microscopic, some of the largest being only about one one-hundred-fiftieth of an inch in diameter. Inside the cyst the amoeba divides until there are, in some cases, as many as eight small parasites instead of one. As this development progresses the cyst passes down the intestine with the feces. By the time it reaches the exterior the development has been completed and the organism is infective to swine.

Swine become infected by swallowing the cysts while feeding on contaminated ground. In the intestine the cyst wall ruptures, releasing the tiny amoebae. Little is known about how long the cysts may remain alive on soil. Since swine often eat fresh feces, however, the infection may be readily acquired in that way.

In severe infections the intestine may become inflamed, and extensive patches of tissue may be destroyed. The parasites burrowing into the wall of the intestine not only erode and destroy patches of tissue but also often rupture small blood vessels which bleed into the intestine. The destruction of the intestinal wall may produce a dysentery in which the feces may be watery and blood-tinged. There is said to be loss of appetite and the infected animal becomes gaunt and has a high fever.

It has been reported that a liquid diet of milk generally brings about a decrease in the numbers of intestinal amoebae in a host.

Balantidia

The balantidia (*Balantidium coli*), though very small in size, are somewhat larger than the amoebae.

When large numbers of balantidia in the active stage are grouped together in water, a trained observer can see them with the unaided eye. In the active stage they have a more or less definite shape, slightly pointed at one end, and are covered with cilia (hairlike structures) by means of which they swim about.

Balantidia are probably the most widespread of the protozoan parasites of pigs, and probably nearly every pig harbours a few of these organisms in its large intestine and blind gut. Considerable difference of opinion exists among investigators as to the actual importance of the parasite as a cause of intestinal disorders in pigs. Some have reported that its presence is frequently associated with severe diarrhoea and even dysentery; others maintain that the parasite does little harm.

Although balantidia ordinarily live in the cavity of the intestine in contact with the cells, they may occasionally invade tissue. They multiply by dividing into equal parts, each part becoming a complete organism. As the feces of the host passes down the intestine, some of the parasites are carried to the exterior. Here some may become round and secrete a heavy cyst wall about themselves, while others die. Some encyst before they pass out with the feces. The cysts vary greatly in size; some may be as large as one-fiftieth of an inch in diameter. Pigs become infected by swallowing the cysts. In the intestine of the pig, the cyst wall is dissolved, and the young parasite emerges and begins to multiply. It has been stated that symptoms of intestinal disorders may appear within 10 to 14 days after infection. A diet rich in starchy grains provides conditions favourable for infection, whereas diets rich in proteins are unfavourable.

It has been observed that suckling pigs may become infected with these protozoa within a few days after birth. The infections may not become noticeable, however, until the pigs are weaned or until they begin to eat solid food. When the pigs are living entirely on milk, the parasites may not pass to the exterior. As soon as the young animal begins to eat grain or other solid food, the parasites may be found in the feces. It has been found possible to free pigs of balantidia by placing the animals on a diet of cow's milk exclusively for about a week. However, an infection does not confer immunity to reinfection.

Occasionally severe intestinal disorders accompany infections of pigs with balantidia, and it has been reported that fat hogs are as a rule the most severely infected. There may be marked depression, loss of appetite, and considerable dysentery, with ulceration and inflammation of the intestine. When present, these symptoms certainly indicate that balantidia may be of considerable importance as a cause of unthriftiness in swine.

Coccidia

Probably the most important protozoan disease of swine is that known as coccidiosis. The disease is caused by the presence in the large intestine of the organisms known as coccidia (*Eimeria*), several species of which occur in pigs. The parasites occur in the cells lining the wall of the intestine, where they grow and develop. In the resistant stages they are called oöcysts. Oöcysts, which correspond to the eggs of worm parasites, are somewhat egg-shaped, and the largest may be about one one-hundredth of an inch in size. They are discharged into the cavity of the intestine, pass out with the droppings, and undergo a period of development before they become infective to swine. Under favourable conditions of moisture and temperature this development is completed in a few days.

Pigs become infected by swallowing the oöcysts while feeding on contaminated ground. Upon reaching the intestine the oöcysts rupture, each releasing several infective bodies. Each of these is capable of penetrating a cell, where it grows at the expense of the cell and produces a number of new infective bodies, which in turn penetrate other cells. Sooner or later some of these bodies develop into oöcysts, which pass out with the droppings and develop to the infective stage.

Owing to the extensive destruction of tissues that normally occurs during the development of the oöcysts, coccidiosis may be a serious disease in pigs, as it usually is in calves and chicks. It has been stated that the pronounced unthriftiness of pigs that commonly occurs on some farms is attributable to coccidia. It is probably the result of the extensive destruction of intestinal cells, which undoubtedly interferes with the absorption of food. According to some investigators, in heavy infections there is a marked thickening of the intestines, which might also interfere with digestion and the absorption of food and water. Experimentally infected pigs lose weight, and the critical stage of the infection lasts about 3 weeks in such pigs.

A characteristic of coccidiosis is that spontaneous recovery may occur. The animal may be severely sick and large numbers of oöcysts may be passing in the feces, when suddenly it begins to get well and the oöcysts disappear. In some cases, however, the disease becomes chronic after it has passed the critical stage, and the pig may remain permanently weak and unthrifty.

Sarcocystis

Sarcocystis miescheriana is a parasite that is considered by some scientists to be related to and by others to be a member of the protozoa. Heavy infections with this organism are characterized by the presence of small white spots in the muscles which may be almost invisible or nearly as large as the head of a pin. In the spots are tiny elongated sacs containing the extremely small spores of the parasite.

Sarcocystis is quite common in garbage-fed hogs; as many as 75 percent of those examined from some localities have been found infected. The parasite is apparently less common in hogs from sections of the country where grain is customarily fed, as only about 5 percent of the animals from these areas have been found on examination to harbour the parasite. The manner in which hogs become infected is unknown, though there have been several theories. Related parasites occur in rats, mice, cattle, sheep, and rabbits.

The flesh of pigs having massive infections with *Sarcocystis* may be light in colour, soft and somewhat watery, and peppered with tiny white spots which are rather indefinite in outline. In older hogs in which the infections are apparently of long standing, the sacs containing the parasites often become greatly enlarged. In many cases the parasites die, and calcification sets in, which produces a gritty condition of the meat. When the lesions of the infection are so large or so numerous as to be visible to the unaided eye, the meat is unfit for food; it is reported that toxic effects have resulted from eating such meat.

Control of Swine Parasites by Treatment

Treatment for the removal of worm parasites is a valuable aid in the control of these pests, especially when combined with sanitary practices designed to prevent reinfection. Removing adult parasites stops the deposition of eggs which sooner or later reach the soil. Moreover, the animal is relieved of the drain caused by parasitic infection. Treatment, however, has certain limitations. Kidney worms and lungworms cannot be removed by the use of drugs, and there are no entirely effective treatments for the removal of whipworms, thorn-headed worms, and intestinal threadworms. Treatments are generally effective against ascarids, nodular worms, and stomach worms, though no single treatment is entirely effective in removing all of them.

For best results, treatment for the removal of parasites should be administered by or under the direction of a veterinarian, since such treatments often involve the administration of drugs that are rather toxic, or poisonous. Drugs that are injurious to the parasite may also be injurious to the pig, and dosages must be properly adjusted. Whether treatment is needed, the kind of medication to use, the proper dosage and method of administration, and whether the physical condition of the animal is such that the drug can be safely administered are matters that involve specialized training.

The drugs recognized to be most effective are oil of chenopodium (wormseed oil), santonin, hexylresorcinol, phenothiazine, and carbon disulfide. The first three are generally effective against adult ascarids in the small intestine. While not entirely satisfactory as a general anthelmintic for swine, phenothiazine in suitable doses is effective in removing nodular worms and moderately effective in removing adult ascarids. Carbon disulfide has been reported to be effective in removing the red stomach worm and has been recommended for the removal of thick stomach worms. The following are approximate dosages of these drugs for animals weighing 100 pounds: Oil of chenopodium, 2 to 4 cubic centimeters; santonin, 1 to 4 grams; hexylresorcinol, 8 grams; carbon disulfide, 8 to 10 cubic centimeters; phenothiazine, 12 grams. The exact dosages, however, must be carefully calculated on the basis of the body weight and physical condition of the animal to be treated.

The four drugs first named may be administered by means of a dose syringe, or stomach tube, or by capsule, following a period of fasting; a purge must be administered at the time of or immediately following administration of the drug. Phenothiazine can be given either in capsules or mixed with four to eight times its weight of dry ground feed without preliminary fasting; no purge is necessary. By using the medicated feed mixture it is possible to treat several pigs at one time.

It should be remembered that treatment alone will not solve the parasite problem. Removal of parasites does not insure against reinfection, and if the animals are kept on contaminated ground the relief afforded by treatment may be only temporary.

Control of Swine Parasites by Management

Management practices designed to break the life cycles of swine parasites at their weakest point, the stage on the ground, are in the long run the cheapest and most effective means of combating these pests.

Two systems have been devised and tested by scientists of the Bureau of Animal Industry. One, called the McLean County system of swine sanitation, was designed for the control of ascarids under conditions prevailing in swine-raising sections of the Midwest. The other, a modification of that system, was designed to control kidney worms under conditions prevailing in the Southeastern States. These systems have for their objects:

(1) The prevention of infection by preventing contact of susceptible animals, as far as possible, with infective stages of the parasites,

(2) The utilization of natural forces in destroying parasite eggs and larvae on soil, and

(3) Simultaneous improvement of the health of the animal through adequate nutrition, since it is recognized that well-fed animals are less likely to become seriously infected than are inadequately fed animals.

The McLean County System of Swine Sanitation

On the basis of the results of investigations on ascarids by scientists in various countries a system of swine sanitation was outlined that would protect pigs from parasite infections during the first few weeks of life (*11*). The plan was then tried out on a practical scale on farms in McLean County, Ill., beginning in the spring of 1920. It was based on the following facts, already brought out in, the discussion of ascarids:

(1) Young pigs are more susceptible to the parasite than older hogs. Pigs suffer most severely from infections during the first few weeks of their lives, becoming more resistant as they grow older.

(2) Pigs become infected by swallowing the infective eggs of the parasite, which occur in the feces of hogs or on the soil of places that have been frequented by hogs.

(3) A single full-grown female worm in the intestine of a hog produces several hundred thousand eggs daily, and as a consequence the soil of areas occupied by infected hogs is likely to be teeming with eggs. The feeding habits of hogs are such that they probably swallow large numbers of eggs daily.

(4) Ascarid eggs are sticky and adhere to the walls and floors of buildings and to the bodies of animals; in these situations they may live for long periods.

(5) Not all adult hogs harbour ascarids even though exposed to infected soil, but the parasites may be found in about one out of every three hogs of breeding age.

Procedures Under the System

It was recognized that in order to protect young pigs against infection it would be necessary to initiate protective measures even before they were born and that from the time of birth to several months of age they would have to be kept entirely away from old hog lots or pastures. The following procedures were therefore devised and tested (*12*):

(1) Clean the farrowing pens thoroughly and then scrub them with scalding water and lye.

Farrowing pens should be of sanitary construction to facilitate cleaning. Shortly before farrowing time the accumulated manure, dirt, and litter should be carefully scraped from the floor, walls, etc., carried away, and either destroyed or plowed under. The entire pen, including walls, floors, guardrails, troughs, etc., should be washed and scrubbed with liberal quantities of very hot water in which lye has been dissolved. If possible, boiling water should be used, for the hotter the water the more effective it will be in destroying parasite eggs. The lye acts as a cleansing agent and helps to remove dirt, in which worm eggs are apt to be lodged.

Recommendations as to the proportion of lye to water vary. Some investigators recommend 1 pound per gallon of water, others 1 pound to 20 gallons. Strong solutions would probably be more effective in removing dirt than would weak solutions. The pen should be scrubbed as the hot lye solution is applied. In the scrubbing, particular attention should be paid to cracks and crevices in floors, walls, troughs, guardrails, and any other places within reach of pigs where parasite eggs may have accumulated. When the pen has been thoroughly scrubbed, it should be rinsed with clean water, and the worker should not reenter the pen; the final rinsing should be accomplished from the outside. The importance of thorough cleansing cannot be overemphasized, as the more thoroughly the job is done the less will be the danger of worm infection.

If there are outside pens in connection with the inside pens, they should also be cleaned if they are of wood or concrete construction; if they have dirt floors, these outside pens should be shut off so as not to be used by the pigs.

If the buildings are not artificially heated, the cleaning should be done in the fall before freezing weather, since it may be difficult to clean properly during cold weather or in early spring or late winter. After being cleaned, the pens should be closed to hogs until farrowing time, and no one should be allowed inside them, as there is always danger of parasite eggs being carried in dirt adhering to shoes.

Cleaning the pens with disinfectants is not recommended, since worm eggs are not killed by most disinfectants.

(2) Clean the sows with warm water and soap just before they are placed in the farrowing pens.

A few days before the sows are due to farrow they should be washed with soap and warm water to remove the mud and dirt that is usually on their skins. Particular attention should be paid to cleaning the udders and sides of the animal where the young pigs will come in close contact with the mother. Immediately after being washed, the sow should be placed in the farrowing pen. It is advisable to wash the sow close to the door of the pen so that she will not have to walk over ground that may be contaminated with worm eggs and thus carry infective material into the pen.

Unless the sows are carefully cleaned before they are placed in the farrowing pens, they may carry with them a multitude of worm eggs and disease germs, so that even within a few hours after the pigs are born they may swallow large numbers of infective agents.

After farrowing, the sows and pigs should not be allowed out of the farrowing pens until they are taken to pasture. Care should be taken by the attendants not to introduce worm eggs into the pens either by entering them wearing dirty shoes or by using dirty troughs or other equipment. Bedding should be changed and the pen cleaned without the attendant entering the pen any more than can be helped.

(3) Haul the pigs and sows from the clean pens to clean pasture. The young pigs and their mothers may be moved to clean pastures any time after warm weather sets in. It is desirable to make the transfer as soon as convenient (within 2 weeks if possible) in order to get the pigs to clean surroundings before the ascarid eggs that may have been deposited by the sow in the pen have reached the infective stage.

The sows and pigs should be hauled, not driven, to the clean pasture. Use of a stone boat with one crate for the sow and another for the pigs is recommended. Some farmers use a double-decked crate with the upper compartment for the pigs and the lower for the sow (Fig. 5). Failure to use caution during the trip from the farrowing house to the pasture may nullify the efforts made in cleaning the sows and pens. A sufficiently large number of worm eggs to cause considerable trouble could be picked up by pigs walking on contaminated ground. An actual example of this was observed by the writer on a farm where a system of sanitation for the control of parasites was being followed. In transferring sows and pigs to a clean pasture the animals were leisurely driven along an old lane for a distance of perhaps 200 yards. This lane had been frequented by hogs at intervals for a period of several years. The majority of the pigs were later found to be infected with ascarids and other parasites.

(4) Keep the young pigs in clean pastures until they are at least 4 months old.

The pasture provided for the sows and pigs should not be a permanent pasture which has recently been used by hogs and may, therefore, be contaminated with worm eggs and larvae. Instead it

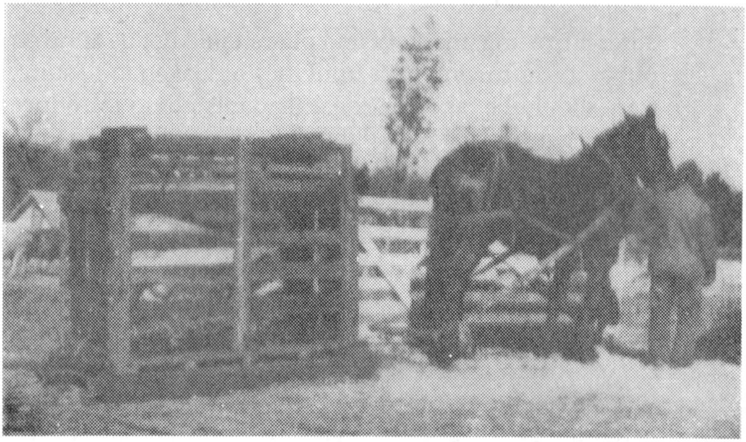

Fig. 5: Hauling the sow and pigs to pasture in a double-decked crate with a space for the sow below and a place for the pigs above. [After Ransom (*12*)].

should be a field that has been under cultivation and sown at the proper time to a suitable forage crop. Legume pastures available in the normal course of crop rotation are desirable, if a different field is devoted to this purpose each year.

In the pasture an individual **A**-type shelter house for each sow and her litter should be provided. This is a small, movable structure built in the form of an **A** with a door at one end. No other hogs should have access to the pasture, and the pigs should not be allowed to run back from the pasture to the barn or lots. If the pigs are thus kept from contaminated places until they are at least 4 months old, there is little likelihood that they will suffer seriously from infections with ascarids. For the best results, however, the animals should be kept away from contaminated areas until they are marketed.

In the case of fall pigs (if not farrowed too late), the same system may be followed with slight modifications. The permanent farrowing house need not be used. If the sows have been on pasture and are not encrusted with dirt and filth, they may be transferred directly to a special temporary pasture and the farrowing may be done in individual **A**-type houses. If the sows have been kept in a hog lot or are encrusted with dirt and filth, they should be washed before being turned into the pasture. In regions not too far north, pigs farrowed by the end of summer will be old enough to be past the ages of greatest susceptibility to ascarid infection before it is necessary to put them into winter quarters that may be more or less contaminated. Even then it is desirable to clean and scrub the hog houses before putting the pigs in them.

Advantages Obtained by Use of the System

When the first practical tests of this system were made on farms, careful records were kept of the number of pigs farrowed, the number of deaths, and the causes of death, together with records of the number of pigs marketed. Following is a summary of reports (*2, 6, 10, 13*) of benefits derived from the use of the system:

(1) More pigs were raised than under the old system of hog raising. In 6 years, on 40 different farms, 6,204 sows farrowed pigs, 39,855 of which were placed on pasture, making an average of 6.4 pigs per litter that survived the farrowing period and reached pasture. Disregarding losses from accidents of various sorts and from hog cholera, the system was 97.8 percent effective in protecting pigs from parasitic and associated hog-lot diseases. Naturally all farmers did not follow the system equally well. On a number of farms where the procedures recommended were closely followed, 1,656 sows farrowed pigs, 10,749 of which reached pasture, an average of 6.5 pigs per litter (*10*).

On the whole, about 76 percent of the pigs farrowed were marketed. Twenty-four percent were lost from all causes, including still-births, accidents, hog cholera, and worms. In contrast, on the farms where the sanitation system was not followed, only about 50 percent of the pigs were marketed (*10*).

(2) Pigs were ready for market earlier.

It was found that pigs raised under the sanitation system were in general ready for market as long as 7 weeks earlier than pigs raised in the ordinary way. It was also found that 4-month-old parasite-free pigs weighed about 28 pounds more on an average than pigs raised on the same farms but not kept under sanitary conditions (*13*).

(3) More pigs were raised per sow.

The system enabled farmers to raise as many pigs as formerly with about two-thirds as many sows. It was estimated (2) that if a farmer needed 17 sows to produce two carloads of 84 or 85 pigs each under ordinary conditions, by using the swine sanitation system he could reduce the number of sows to 12. The cost of feed necessary to maintain 5 sows, estimated to be about $30 per sow per year, could thus be saved.

The effectiveness of the swine sanitation system in saving pigs is further illustrated by the following report (*6*): A group of 12 sows farrowed 117 pigs in an old hog lot. Parasitism and other hog-lot diseases reduced the number until only 35 pigs remained to be marketed. The following year the same 12 sows farrowed 95 pigs. By following the programme of good feeding, good housing, and clean pastures, 90 of these pigs were raised to market weight.

The fact needs emphasis that if maximum benefit is to be derived from swine sanitation the entire procedure must be followed closely, as lack of thoroughness in any step results in a corresponding decline in effectiveness (*1*). It was observed, for example, that of a group of 160 farmers those who merely cleaned but did not scrub farrowing pens before the sows were put in them raised an average of 5.05 pigs per litter. Those who both cleaned and scrubbed pens raised an average of 5.67 pigs per litter. Still others who cleaned and washed the farrowing pens and also washed the sows raised an average of 6.85 pigs per litter. The owners who followed all these steps and in addition transferred the pigs to clean pastures during the suckling period raised an average of 8 pigs per litter.

An important aspect of parasite control in pigs, which is of ten overlooked or disregarded by the farmer but which materially increases the effectiveness of any control measure, is the matter of a well-balanced diet provided in adequate amounts for the growing animals. Ordinarily the full-fed pig is the healthiest pig. For one thing, it has more of the vitality necessary to resist or throw off disease agents than a pig on a deficient or inadequate diet. Also the adequacy and sufficiency of the diet have a marked effect on the feeding habits of the pigs, and this in turn directly influences the extent, of the parasite infections acquired. Pigs full-fed from self-feeders are less likely to become seriously infected with parasites than scantily fed pigs or pigs fed from ground where the feed comes in contact with feces. Inadequately fed pigs spend much time searching for food on the ground, where it is generally contaminated with agents of disease.

The part that feeding habits may play in parasite infection is indicated by the following observations made in connection with nodular worm infections of pigs on two farms where a system for the control of parasites was being tested (*18*):

On one farm the recommendations were carefully followed except that insufficient feed was made available to the pigs. As a result the animals were constantly hungry and spent a large part of their time rooting and searching for food on ground contaminated with the feces of the sows, which were infected with nodular worms. The pigs were frequently seen eating grains of corn that had passed undigested in the feces of the sows. Examination of such feces and the surrounding soil invariably revealed the presence of infective larvae of nodular worms. At slaughter the intestines of the pigs were found studded with nodules and harbouring hundreds of nodular worms.

On the other farm, where the recommended procedures were followed and in addition adequate amounts of a well-balanced diet were made constantly available in self-feeders, the pigs spent little time in rooting and searching for food on the ground. After eating from the self-feeders, the pigs would lie down in the shade until they were hungry again. They were never seen to eat corn passed in the feces of the sows. When slaughtered, the majority of the pigs were found to be free of nodular worms, and the remainder were only slightly infected. In spite of the fact that these animals had as much opportunity as the underfed pigs to become infected with nodular worms, the infections acquired were relatively unimportant owing to their feeding habits.

The influence of adequate nutrition on infection with internal parasites applies also to very young pigs. Young pigs whose mothers do not provide adequate milk soon begin rooting and searching for food on the ground, from which they are likely to acquire infection with parasites, especially those having direct life histories. It has been observed that litters of pigs farrowed in old hog lots by sows that did not provide adequate nourishment for their offspring became infected with parasites during the first few days of their existence. In contrast, some of the pigs farrowed in the same lot by sows that provided adequate milk for their pigs did not become infected for several weeks, and some did not become infected at all during the period they were kept under observation (*21*).

The observations related show that in addition to the recommended procedures for the control of parasites in pigs, two additional precautions can be taken by the farmer which may aid materially in controlling these pests:

(1) Select sows for breeding that provide adequate milk for the suckling pigs, especially during the early stages of lactation; in other words, use only sows that are good milkers

(2) As soon as the pigs begin to eat, provide adequate amounts of a well-balanced diet in self-feeders.

Kidney Worm Control Plan

Because kidney worms cannot be removed from the body of the living animal by the use of drugs, it was early recognized that the only way to cope with this parasite was to prevent infection. Although various measures for controlling kidney worms had already been recommended, none was entirely applicable to conditions in the United States. An investigation was therefore begun to ascertain the factors responsible for the spread of kidney worms, such as:

(1) The distribution and length of survival of the larvae on pastures,

(2) The effect of climatic factors on the eggs and larvae, and

(3) The conditions under which pigs acquire infection. The investigation was carried out under actual field conditions in one of the Southern States where kidney worms constitute a serious problem, and the following facts were ascertained (*19*):

    (1) Infective kidney worm larvae are most abundant in and beneath trash and litter, such as corn husks, etc., that accumulate on feeding grounds. The larvae also occur in lesser numbers on the soil of moist, shaded areas, along fences, under trees, and in and around hog houses and other buildings frequented by hogs. The larvae are widely distributed over pastures where the grass is dense enough to shade the ground and thus retains a certain amount of moisture around the

roots. Infective larvae are not common in wallows and do not live long under such conditions.

(2) On soil where they are protected from direct sunlight, drying, and freezing temperatures, kidney worm larvae may persist for 3 months or longer.

(3) Kidney worm larvae are very sensitive to the effects of direct sunlight, under which they fail to survive more than 1 hour even when not subjected also to drying.

(4) Kidney worm eggs deposited by infected animals on unshaded bare soil live only a few hours on sunshiny days. Under these conditions the eggs are apparently killed by the combined effects of the sunlight and drying.

(5) The greatest concentrations of kidney worm eggs occur on the soil beneath accumulated trash and litter on the feeding ground, on soil in the vicinity of farrowing houses and shelters, and on paths along the fences that surround the pasture. It was observed that on waking and leaving the shelters sows would generally urinate after walking a short distance, thereby contributing to the concentration of eggs on the soil near the farrowing houses and shelters.

(6) The infective larvae may migrate from the soil up the stems and blades of grass at night when the vegetation is wet with dew. As the sun comes up and the grass begins to dry, many of the larvae return to the damp, shaded portions of the grass and to the soil beneath.

(7) Infective larvae are stimulated by moderate heat and will migrate short distances toward a warmer environment.

On the basis of these facts and observations of the habits of swine and of husbandry practices in common use in the region where kidney worms are abundant, a plan of management for sows and litters that has for its object the protection of pigs from infection with kidney worms while they are with the sow was devised (*19*). The objective is accomplished by the use of temporary pastures and a simple arrangement of farrowing equipment (**A**-type houses, feeding and watering devices, etc.) in relation to the pasture areas so as to take advantage of various climatic factors to insure destruction of the eggs and larvae of kidney worms.

Figure 6 is a photograph of a model of a kidney worm control set-up. The arrangement of equipment shown was designed to insure, as far as possible, that the majority of the kidney worm eggs passed by the sows will fall on places where they cannot survive. It provides under actual farm conditions an effective means of breaking the life cycle of the parasite at its weakest point, the stage on the ground. Tests carried out on farms in the kidney worm belt have

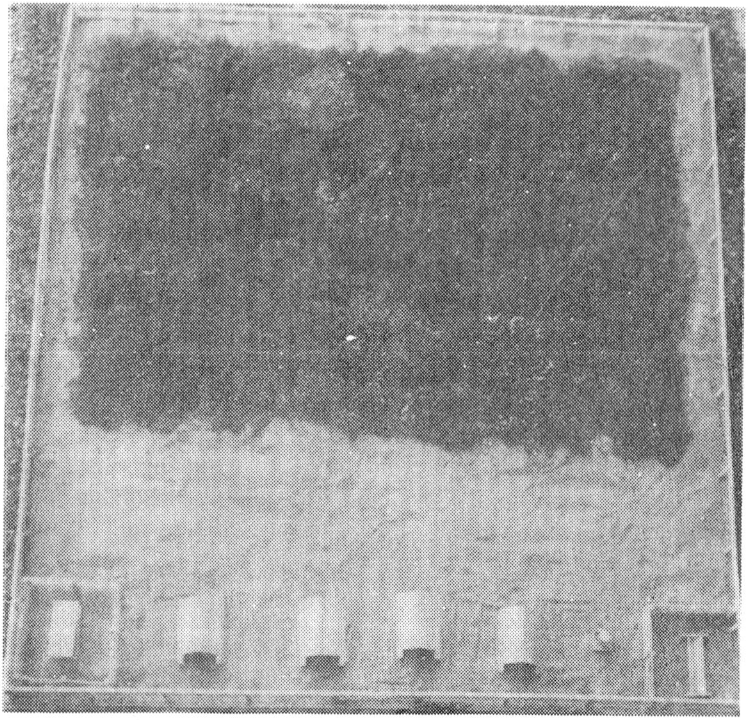

Fig. 6: A model set-up for kidney worm control. At the bottom, close to and facing the fence, are four A-type farrowing houses. Also on the bare area are a creep for the pigs (left-hand corner), a feeding pen for the sows (right-hand corner), and a watering barrel.

shown this arrangement to be an effective control measure. The bare area must, however, be kept free of trash and vegetation of all kinds.

The sequence of steps to be followed in carrying out this plan has been outlined in detail elsewhere (*15*), but they will be enumerated and briefly discussed here.

(1) Put pregnant sows shortly before farrowing on a pasture that has been especially prepared by being sown to a suitable forage crop.

Temporary pastures of oats, rye, or some other suitable crop should always be utilized for this purpose. The area should be one that has been plowed and had at least one crop grown on it since last being used by hogs. This precaution is to insure destruction of kidney worm larvae and the infective stages of many other parasites.

(2) In sowing, leave an area of bare soil all around the pasture.

The bare area should be about 5 feet wide on each of three sides of the pasture and at least 30 feet wide at one end (Fig. 6). The wider portion is to accommodate the farrowing or shelter houses, water barrel, creep for pigs, and feeding pen for sows. The wide area should be at the end of the field most convenient for taking care of the animals without having to cross the entire field.

(3) Keep the bare portions of the field free of all trash, litter, and vegetation.

If trash is allowed to accumulate and grass to grow on the bare area, the purpose of the plan may be defeated, since such accumulations provide protection for the larvae. It may be necessary to cultivate the bare areas from time to time, using a plow disk or some other implement to destroy grass that may start up. The parasite eggs deposited by the sows around the houses and during the course of their wanderings along fence rows will thus be exposed to sunlight and drying, the farmer's best allies in combating parasites.

(4) A creep large enough for the pigs should be located on the bare area and not in the pasture area.

It is essential that the creep be located on the bare area and that the area surrounding it be kept free of trash and vegetation. This is necessary because sows often remain in the vicinity of the creep when the pigs are feeding and contaminate the surrounding soil with their urine and feces. When the creep is located on the pasture area it has been found that the accumulation of kidney worm larvae around it constitutes a source of infection for the pigs. When the creep is on bare soil, the eggs will be destroyed and will not be important in the spread of kidney worms except during long spells of damp, cloudy weather.

(5) The feeding pen for the sows should be located some distance away from the creep.

It has been found advantageous from the standpoint of parasite control to feed the sows in a separate pen. The pen should be so arranged that the pigs cannot have access to it at any time. The sows should be fed in the pen and should be allowed to remain there for some time after feeding so that they may urinate and defecate where the pigs will not have access to the infective material.

(6) A watering barrel of sanitary construction should be located on the bare strip.

The arrangement should be such that the barrel will not overflow and thus create a wet area around it that might be favourable for the survival of parasite eggs and larvae.

(7) An **A**-type farrowing house should be provided for each sow.

The farrowing houses should be located on the bare strip at a distance of about 6 feet from and facing the fence. The houses should be placed some distance apart. Trash and litter, such as bedding, should not be allowed to accumulate around the houses to provide shelter for kidney worms. It has been found that larvae of nodular worms often occur inside farrowing houses and beneath shelters in small particles of fecal material carried in on the bodies and feet of the animals. The bedding inside the houses should therefore be changed from time to time in order to remove fecal material that may have been tracked in.

Control of kidney worms is accomplished by this procedure in the following ways:

(1) Since the sows usually urinate not far from their shelter houses (especially after waking), near fences, and near the creep, the kidney worm eggs they excrete fall on soil that remains bare and dry (except during wet seasons) and are destroyed by sunlight and drying. Although the sows frequently urinate while grazing on the pasture area, the eggs are generally so scattered as to reduce the chances of infection materially.

(2) The use of a separate feeding pen for the sows, to which the pigs are never admitted and where the sows are left for a time after feeding, assures that many worm eggs will be concentrated in a location inaccessible to the pigs. Better results may be obtained if the manure is removed from the feeding pen at frequent intervals and disposed of so that the pigs will not come in contact with it.

Feeding the sows in a separate pen is desirable from another standpoint. During the gestation and lactation period, it makes it possible to exercise some control over the diet of the sow with a minimum amount of trouble.

Results Obtained by Use of the System

As a measure of the effect of these management practices in controlling kidney worms, careful post mortem examinations have been made from time to time of swine raised in accordance with the procedures recommended. Examinations were recently made of 525 pigs raised by this plan on farms in southern Georgia and northern Florida. Slight kidney worm lesions were present in the kidneys of only 10 percent of the animals. Only 14 percent of the livers were condemned as unfit for food because of these parasites. Naturally some of the farmers had not adhered strictly to the prescribed plan, and consequently some of the animals became infected. In 21 herds that were raised strictly in accordance with the provisions recommended, all livers were passed for food and the kidneys and kidney fat of all the animals were free of worms.

In marked contrast to those results, in 53,000 hogs raised without any attempt to prevent infection, 92 percent of the livers and all the kidneys and kidney fat were found parasitized with kidney worms and were condemned as unfit for food (*15*).

Other benefits derived from the kidney worm control plan include the raising of more pigs, better and more economical gains, and consequently more profit. Information gleaned from reports of county agents, directors of 4-H Clubs, and extension workers shows that by following the system in its entirety many farmers save more of their pigs and the young animals grow faster than under the old system. According to reports, some farmers have been able to market pigs anywhere from several weeks to as long as 3 months earlier than was customary. For example, it is reported that where the system has been carefully followed and the pigs were force-fed, it has been possible to market them at 200 pounds live weight in 5 months. It has also been stated that pigs grow more uniformly than when raised without attention to sanitation, and that hogs raised free from kidney worms and other parasites often dress out better than wormy hogs. In some cases the carcasses of the worm-free animals have dressed out over 78 percent. The difference is illustrated in figure 3, which shows the carcasses of a worm-free and a wormy hog, each 6 months of age.

Some criticism of the system has been made on the ground that it entails some trouble and expense. Practically the only unusual expense is that of providing shelter houses, water barrels, and feeding pens. However, these need not be elaborate structures and can be built of materials already on the farm. Once constructed, they can be used for many years.

As for the extra effort the system entails, if a farmer depends for part of his income on profit from the hogs he raises, he should consider the raising of the animals as an integral part of his farm programme and give as much attention to it as he would to the corn, cotton, peanuts, and other crops he grows. It is well recognized that certain types of land are unsuited for growing grain, forage, or other plant crops and that any attempt to grow these crops on such soil would meet with failure. It should likewise be recognized that certain types of locations, such as permanent pastures, low-lying areas, etc., are unsuited for growing a pig crop. Any attempt to utilize such lands for pigs is likely to meet with partial or complete failure to raise the crop at a profit.

The farmer fights diseases and insects that affect his grain, forage, and fiber crops, and he fertilizes the soil to provide adequate nourishment for the plants to promote maximum growth. The pig crop is no different. The pigs have diseases that should be combated and need adequate nourishment to promote good health and maximum growth.

Pigs cannot be raised successfully on wasteland without attention any more than peanuts or corn can be expected to thrive on swampy or stony ground without proper attention. The farmer who wants to make a profit from his hogs should devote some of his best land to that purpose each year, just as he would to a plant crop on which he expects to make money. The pig crop should receive as careful attention as the plant crop, and it will not only give maximum returns but will also pay extra dividends by enriching the soil.

Literature Cited

(1) ANONYMOUS (1926). SWINE SANITATION. (Abstract) Vet. Med. 21: 501.

(2) BURCH, J.W. (1930). THE MISSOURI PLAN OF GROWING THRIFTY PIGS. Mo. Univ. Agr. Col. Cir. 259, 12 pp., illus.

(3) CLUNIES ROSS, I., and KAUZAL, G. (1932). THE LIFE CYCLE OF STEPHANURUS DENTATUS DEISING, 1839: THE KIDNEY WORM OF PIGS. WITH OBSERVATIONS ON ITS ECONOMIC IMPORTANCE IN AUSTRALIA AND SUGGESTIONS FOR ITS CONTROL. Austral. Council Sci. & Indus. Res., Bul. 58, 80 pp., illus.

(4) CRAM, ELOISE B. (1930). BIRDS AS A FACTOR IN THE CONTROL OF A STOMACH WORM OF SWINE. Auk (n.s.) 47: 380-384.

(5) FRANCIONI, J.B., and MORRIS, HARRY (1930). IT PAYS TO TREAT PIGS FOB WORMS. La. State Univ. Ext. Cir. 96, 10 pp., illus. (Revised).

(6) GIBSON, J.E. (1931). SWINE-SANITATION PLAN RESULTS IN MORE AND BETTER PIGS PER SOW. U.S. Dept. Agr. Yearbook 1931: 503-505, illus.

(7) KATES, K.C. (1941). OBSERVATIONS ON THE VIABILITY OF EGGS OF LUNGWORMS OF SWINE. Jour. Parasitol. 27: 265-272.

(8) NIGHBERT, E.M., and CONNELLY, J.W. (1928). LOSSES THROUGH CONDEMNATIONS DUE TO PARASITES AND PARASITIC CONDITIONS OF SWINE, AND THE EFFECT OF SWINE SANITATION IN THE CONTROL OF KIDNEY WORMS. [Privately printed cir., Swift and Co.], [6] pp.

(9) PRICE, EMMETT W. (1925). THE OCCURRENCE AND DISTRIBUTION OF CYSTICERCUS CELLULOSAE IN TEXAS SWINE. Jour. Parasitol. 12: [81]-83, illus.

(10) RAFFENSPERGER, H.B., and CONNELLY, J.W. (1927). THE SWINE SANITATION SYSTEM AS DEVELOPED BY THE BUREAU OF ANIMAL

INDUSTRY IN M'LEAN COUNTY, ILL. U.S. Dept. Agr. Tech. Bul. 44, 20 pp.

(11) RANSOM, B.H. (1918). WORKS IN PIGS. U.S. Dept. Agr. Weekly News Letter 5 (35): 5.

(12) _____(1927). THE PREVENTION OF ROUNDWORMS IN PIGS. U.S. Dept. Agr. Leaflet 6, 8 pp., illus.

(13) ROBBINS, E.T. (1926). CHEAPER AND MORE PROFITABLE PORK THRU SWINE SANITATION. A REVIEW OF THE M'LEAN COUNTY SYSTEM OF SWINE SANITATION ON ILLINOIS FARMS DURING 1925. Ill. Agr. Expt. Sta. Cir. 306, 16 pp., illus.

(14) SCHWARTZ, BENJAMIN (1931). SWINE KIDNEY WORM CAUSES LOSS TO SOUTHERN PRODUCERS FROM CONDEMNED CARCASSES. U.S. Dept. Agr. Yearbook 1931: 499-502, illus.

(15) _____(1934). CONTROLLING KIDNEY WORMS IN SWINE IN THE SOUTHERN STATES. U.S. Dept. Agr. Leaflet 108, 6 pp., illus.

(16) _____and PRICE, E.W. (1929). THE LIFE HISTORY OF THE SWINE KIDNEY WORM. Science 70: 613-614.

(17) SHOPE, RICHARD E. (1939). AN INTERMEDIATE HOST FOR THE SWINE INFLUENZA VIRUS. Science 89: 441-442.

(18) SPINDLER, L.A. (1933). FIELD STUDIES OF THE LARVAE OF NODULAR WORMS OF SWINE, WITH SUGGESTIONS FOR CONTROL. North Amer. Vet. 14 (11): 37-44.

(19) _____(1934). FIELD AND LABORATORY STUDIES ON THE BEHAVIOUR OF THE LARVAE OF THE SWINE KIDNEY WORM, STEPHANURUS DENTATUS. U.S. Dept. Agr. Tech. Bul. 405, 18 pp.

(20) _____(1934). SKIN PENETRATION EXPERIMENTS WITH THE INFECTIVE LARVAE OF STEPHANURUS DENTATUS. North Amer. Vet. 15 (10): 32-36.

(21) _____(1937). INFESTATION OF SUCKLING PIGS WITH HELMINTH PARASITES UNDER CONDITION OF CONSTANT EXPOSURE TO INFECTION. Helminthol. Soc. Wash. Proc. 4: 62-63.

(22) _____(1938). PERSISTENCE OF SWINE LUNGWORM LARVAE IN EARTHWORMS. Helminthol. Soc. Wash. Proc. 5: 63.

Chapter 10

TRICHINOSIS

Benjamin Schwartz[1]

[1] *Benjamin Schwartz is Chief of the Zoological Division, Bureau of Animal Industry.*

Recent surveys show that far more people in the United States are infected with trichinae–the small worms that settle chiefly in the muscles and cause trichinosis–than was formerly thought to be the case. Human beings get the disease almost entirely from pork. It can be prevented by the methods-described in this article.

The microscopic roundworm parasites that occur at times in the muscles of human beings, swine, dogs, cats, rats, mice, and many other omnivorous and carnivorous animals are known to the general public as trichinae and to biologists and medical scientists as *Trichinella spiralis*. These parasites, when present in sufficient numbers in a suitable host, produce a disease known as trichinosis or trichiniasis.

Although trichinosis is probably never diagnosed in swine and seldom in other animals during life, the disease as it appears in man presents a more or less definite chain of symptoms, principally fever, muscular pains, and swelling of the eyelids. It may terminate in death and, in fact, is known to produce fatal results in about 5 percent of the cases. Because infected pork eaten raw or imperfectly cooked is the main source of human trichinosis, the occurrence of trichinae in swine has a far greater significance as a possible hazard to human health than as a cause of sickness in the affected animals.

In the discussion that follows trichinae are considered, therefore, iargely as a menace to human health. The public health aspect of swine trichinosis, which has been widely publicized in recent years, has produce considerable repercussions in this country to the detriment of swine producers and the meat industry.

The Discovery that Trichinae Produce Disease

Trichinae were named and described in 1835, a quarter of a century before they were shown definitely to have any influence on human and animal health. There is some reason to believe that these parasites were actually observed in England in 1822 and again in 1828. In fact it appears quite certain that trichinae in their cysts, or capsules, were found in England by Hilton in 1832 in the abdominal muscles of a human cadaver. Hilton, who was a demonstrator in anatomy in Guy's Hospital, London, did not investigate the contents of these cysts, and the credit for doing this for the first time belongs to his fellow countryman, Paget, who made his observations 3 years later. In 1835 Paget, a medical student, discovered, while dissecting the muscles of a human body, small gritty spots that took the keen edge off his scalpel. Fortunately he had enough curiosity to investigate these spots with the aid of a microscope and, with technical assistance from others, determined that the spots were actually cysts containing organisms. He turned the material over to his professor, Sir Richard Owen, who in the same year published an account (*10*)[2] of the encysted parasites now known as *Trichinella spiralis*.

Following their discovery, trichinae, later recognized to roundworms, continued to be encountered from time to time in dissecting rooms and for the next 25 years were regarded by most medical workers as relatively harmless zoological curiosities. The discovery by Leidy of trichinae in pork in the United States in 1846 (*6*) and a similar discovery in a cat in Germany some time later apparently threw no light on the possible origin of these muscle parasites. How they got into the muscles and how they propagated

[2] Italic numbers in parentheses refer to Literature Cited.

remained a complete mystery for two and one-half decades following their discovery, though speculation on these points was not lacking.

Like some other important discoveries in parasitology, those relating to trichinae were begun with simple observations that were followed later by experiments to determine the essential facts in the life cycle. In 1851 Herbst published an account of experiments in which he fed to dogs meat from a badger that, presumably, had been infected experimentally with trichinae; some time later he discovered encysted trichinae in the dogs' muscles. Investigations carried out in Germany a few years later by Leuckart, Zenker, and Virchow demonstrated conclusively that trichinae in the muscles of man and animals are actually incompletely developed worms, distinct from all others known up to that time as parasites of man and animals, and capable of undergoing further growth and development in the intestines of suitable hosts. Finally, these three investigators working at the same time but independently, elucidated the essential facts in the mode of transmission of trichinae and established beyond doubt that the worms that occur in the muscles are the infective stages of parasites that can grow to maturity in the intestines of susceptible host animals that have ingested trichina-infected meat.

That pork is a source of human infection came to light in 1860 under rather dramatic circumstances:

While conducting a necropsy, or post mortem examination, on a 19-year-old girl who died in Dresden, Germany, early in 1860, of a disease that was diagnosed before her death as typhoid fever, Zenker failed to find the usual post mortem picture characteristic of that disease. He found, however, numerous unencysted trichinae in the girl's muscles. Part of this material he sent to Leuckart and part to Virchow, the former an outstanding zoologist and parasitologist and the latter known the world over as the founder of cellular pathology. These investigators determined by animal experimentation that the trichinae found in the muscles of the girl developed to maturity in the intestines of suitable hosts, the mature parasites, in turn, evidently producing a new generation of young worms that ultimately invaded the muscles. Meanwhile Zenker discovered mature trichinae in the girl's intestines. He learned, moreover, that she had eaten raw sausage a month or so before her death. Fortunately some of the sausage was still available in the household where she had been a servant, and an examination showed that it was heavily infected with trichinae. Moreover, Zenker elicited the information that others in the household who had eaten this sausage had also become sick.

Thus in the year 1860 trichinae were shown to be pathogenic (disease producing) to man and capable of causing death; infected pork was shown to be a source of human trichinosis; and the mode of transmission of trichinae from one animal to another was conclusively established by rigid scientific experimentation. Perhaps the strongest occurrence in the unraveling of the story of trichinosis was the demonstration by Leuckart and Virchow, on the same day but quite independently of one another (*8*), of the presence of unencysted trichinae in the muscles of test animals to which infected meat had been fed several weeks earlier. The unencysted worms which Leuckart found in the muscles of an experimentally infected hog and Virchow found in those of an experimentally infected rabbit were in the same stage of development as those found by Zenker in the muscles of the girl whose death was the first to be definitely recorded in medical literature as due to human trichinosis.

Life History of Trichinae

The life history of trichinae is shown graphically in Fig. 1. It is evident that infection results from eating meat that harbours trichinae. As a rule, human beings acquire trichinae by eating raw or imperfectly cooked trichinous pork in one form or another; swine become infected by eating offal or garbage containing scraps of raw infected pork or by eating the flesh of infected rats, mice, or other animals (Fig. 1, sec. 5); rats and mice, in turn, acquire trichinae by eating raw, trichina-infected pork or other infected meat in garbage or elsewhere, or through cannibalism; dogs, cats, and other carnivorous animals acquire these parasites by eating the flesh of other animals already infected. Regardless of the source of infection, the course of events following the consumption of trichinous meat is briefly as follows:

As the trichina-infected meat is digested in the stomach of a human being, hog, or other suitable host, the encapsulated worms (Fig. 1, sec. 4), are freed from their lemon-shaped or spherical capsules, or cysts, which are approximately one-fiftieth of an inch in maximum diameter and therefore microscopic in size. The worms themselves, spirally coiled within the cyst, are cylindrical in shape and measure about one twenty-fifth of an inch from end to end. Once they are free in the cavity, or lumen, of the stomach, they pass rapidly into the small intestine and become localized among the folds and villi (minute projections of the inner lining). Here they increase in size and attain sexual maturity in 2 days or earlier (3). Following the mating of the sexes, the worms continue to grow, and they attain their maximum size 4 to 5 days later, or 6 to 7 days after they reach the host's stomach. When full grown, the females measure from one-eighth to one-sixth of an inch in length; the males are only about half as long (Fig. 1, sec. 1). The fertilized eggs are not discharged by the female worms, as are those of most other parasitic roundworms that occur in man and domestic animals, but develop within the maternal uterus, where they hatch and from which they escape as larvae.

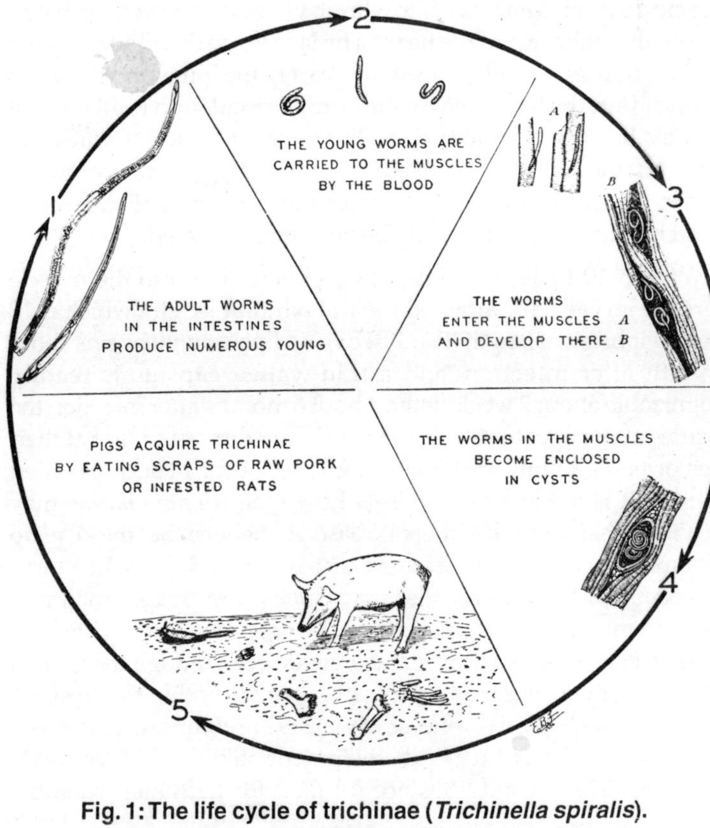

Fig. 1: The life cycle of trichinae (*Trichinella spiralis*).

The birth of the larvae begins about 5 days after infection (*3*) and may continue for several weeks; though many more young are born during the first 2 weeks of the worms' fertile period than subsequently. The adult trichinae in the intestine tend to die and pass out after their reproductive functions have been fulfilled, though adult worms have been found several weeks after infection and some of them, at least, may persist for 3 months or so. The newborn larvae (Fig. 1, sec. 2), of which several hundred can be deposited by a single female trichina (*9*), measure about one two hundred and fiftieth of an inch in length. Owing to the fact that the female worm is rather deeply imbedded in the intestinal lining, the larvae are deposited directly in the lymph spaces of the intestinal wall. The larvae thus caught in the lymph channels migrate with the lymph stream, ultimately reaching one of the large lymph vessels, known as the thoracic duct. This empties into a large vein, from which the blood flows to the right side of the heart. The larvae are distributed by the circulation from the right side of the heart to the lungs and thence to the left side of the heart and by the arterial circulation to all parts of the body. It is known that trichina larvae reach various tissues and organs but they become localized, for the most part, in the voluntary muscles (the flesh), the fibers of which they penetrate (Fig. 1, sec. 3, *A*) and in which they ultimately become encapsulated.

Within 10 to 14 days after their penetration into the muscle fibers the larvae have attained their maximum length, which is 10 times their original length (Fig. 1, sec. 3, *B*). Encystment begins about 1 month after infection, and a thin-walled capsule is readily recognizable about 2 weeks later. About 6 months after infection the capsules may begin to calcify, calcium being deposited first at their poles or ends. Living trichinae commonly occur in such calcified capsules. It is not known precisely how long trichina larvae may live within their cysts, but there is reason to believe that they can do so for many years, at least in some cases. Sooner or later, however, the worms within the capsules may calcify and break down into crumbled masses, or they may die before the process of calcification has set in and become absorbed. However, even though the worms remain alive they are incapable of further growth within the capsules. In many respects the live, encysted worms are comparable to seeds which are capable of further development only under favourable conditions. These conditions are fulfilled for trichinae when the flesh, or meat, in which they are present is eaten by an animal in which they are capable of developing to sexual maturity, as previously described.

Hosts of Trichinae

Trichinae have been recorded from a variety of animals besides those mentioned. Bears, in particular, can play an important role in the transmission of trichinae to man, severe cases of this infection in Europe having been traced to the eating of uncooked bear meat. In the United States there have been instances in which jerked bear meat has been found to be a source of human trichinosis. Various other carnivorous animals, such as the fox, the badger, the martin, the raccoon, the otter, the mongoose, and others are known to be hosts of trichinae. Several wild rodents, such as the mole, the hedgehog, the ground squirrel, and others, also have been reported as hosts of these parasites. In the laboratory, rabbits, guinea pigs, white rats, and mice are readily infected experimentally with trichinae, and much of the available information about these parasites is a result of the experimental infection of these rodents. The herbivorous domestic animals–cattle, sheep, goats, and horses–also are susceptible to experimental infection with trichinae. Under normal conditions, however, these animals would not become infected, since they do not eat meat, and so far as is known, their susceptibility is only of theoretical interest and without any practical significance.

In certain European countries the flesh of various fur-bearing animals, in addition to that of bears, is sometimes eaten raw or incompletely cooked, with the result that some cases of human trichinosis have been traced to this source. In the United States, however, all cases of trichinosis that have been definitely traced to their source, with the exception of a few known to have resulted from eating uncooked bear meat, were found to have been caused by the eating of raw or rare pork or some pork-containing meat food product, such as sausage, insufficiently processed to destroy trichinae. Cases of trichinosis usually occur after parties, picnics, and family gatherings in which raw ham or sausage or some other insufficiently cooked or inadequately cured pork-containing food is eaten by relatively large groups, only those who abstain from eating the food in question escaping infection (*16*).

The Disease

Symptoms

The disease trichinosis manifests itself in man and animals by various symptoms, the severity of which is usually correlated with the number of worms swallowed in the infected meat. The consumption of lightly infected pork or other meat by man or animals produces no visible symptoms unless large quantities of such meat are eaten. On the other hand, the consumption of even relatively small quantities of heavily infected meat may produce serious illness and even death.

The clinical manifestations of trichinosis in swine have been established by experimental feeding of large quantities of trichinous meat. In the severest cases intestinal irritation, fever, muscular pain and stiffness, difficulty in chewing and breathing, and severe emaciation have been noted. In more moderate infections the symptoms are indefinite. Trichinosis in pigs is not diagnosed during the life of these animals, even though the symptoms are striking, for the reason that other, more familiar febrile diseases–that is, diseases accompanied by fever–of swine are characterized by similar clinical manifestations.

In man the clinical picture of trichinosis has been ascertained in various parts of the world since 1860. The classical accounts of this disease as recorded in the medical literature are briefly as follows:

During the development of trichinae in the intestine and the production of their young, known as the stage of ingression, there may be nausea, vomiting, diarrhoea, and abdominal pain, or these symptoms may be entirely lacking. Other manifestations during the first week or so of infection are a general torpor, accompanied by weakness, a sensation of tension or pain in the muscles, muscular twitching, and, towards the end of this period, a swelling of the face and eyelids, particularly the latter.

The next stage of the disease, known as the stage of digression, corresponds to the distribution of the larvae throughout the body and their penetration into the muscles. The symptoms of this stage appear after the first week, about 9 days to 2 weeks after initial infection, and continue for the next 2 weeks or so. They are characterized by severe muscular pains, the muscles becoming swollen, hard, and tense. Moving the eyes and the tongue and chewing, breathing, swallowing are likely to be painful because of the penetration of trichina larvae.

The third stage, known as the stage of regression, corresponds to the encystment of the parasites within the muscles and may be accompanied by an intensification of the symptoms of the second stage and the appearance of pronounced swelling of the legs, forearms, abdominal wall, and face. Anemia and cutaneous (skin) eruptions may appear, and pneumonia is a probable complication.

Fever sets in during the first stage, becomes more pronounced during the second stage, and may persist, usually with remissions, for several weeks. Apathy or mental disturbances may set in, and in some cases the mental symptoms may become aggravated to the point of delirium.

The symptoms outlined represent, no doubt, a composite picture of the disease. All of them would not be present in all cases, nor would they appear necessarily in the order mentioned. Actually the clinical picture may show striking variations, as indicated in accounts of a recent outbreak of trichinosis in England (*5, 20*) involving about 500 clinical and an undetermined number of subclinical cases.

Diagnosis

In a few cases practicing veterinarians have diagnosed trichinosis in pet animals, largely on the basis of fever associated with muscular stiffness. In man a presumptive diagnosis of trichinosis is frequently made on the basis of symptoms, particularly if the clinical manifestations can be traced to the consumption of raw pork or some pork, food product not sufficiently processed to destroy trichinae. Not infrequently, however, the clinical manifestations of trichinosis in man have been confused with those of other febrile diseases, especially typhoid fever, undulant fever, influenza, nephritis, tuberculous meningitis, gastroenteritis, colitis, rheumatic endocarditis, syphilis, tuberculosis, and other diseases.

Of the more important diagnostic aids that are used to corroborate a presumptive diagnosis of trichinosis, eosinophilia (an increase in certain white blood cells–the eosinophilic leucocytes of the blood), a positive skin test and blood serum test, and the discovery of trichinae in small pieces of muscle (biopsy material), are the most important.

Incidence of Trichinae and of Trichinosis in Man

Investigations conducted in the United States during the last 12 years and still in progress have disclosed a surprisingly high incidence of infection with trichinae in the general population of this country. The investigations under consideration have been conducted by means of one or both of two techniques:

(1) Digesting, in an incubator, the diaphragm or other muscle tissues, or sizable portions of them, obtained from the bodies of persons that have died in hospitals from various causes other than trichinosis, and recovering any trichinae present from the sediment of the digestive fluid;

(2) Repeated, painstaking microscopic examinations of fresh preparations of diaphragm or other muscle tissue in which trichinae are known to be localized in large numbers.

Queen (*11*) reported in 1931 that the muscle samples from 59 of 344 unselected persons (17.2 percent) who died in Rochester, N.Y., and those from 16 of 58 persons (27.6 percent) who died in Boston, Mass., contained trichinae; other investigators working in or obtaining their material for the most part from large metropolitan hospitals afterward published more or less similar results. In some of these cases the reported incidences of infection with trichinae were even more striking than those recorded by queen. A recent report issued by the United States Public Health Service (*4*) covers the examination for trichinae of 2,330 human diaphragms obtained from hospitals in Washington, D.C., and 670 from various Federal hospitals in other cities. Of the total number examined, 488 (16.3 percent) were infected with trichinae. It is important to note, however, that 425 contained trichinae in rather small numbers, probably too few, in most cases, to have produced any signs of illness during life. Only 8 of the 488 positive diaphragms contained more than 100 larvae per gram of muscle tissue examined, and it is not unlikely that these were from the only individuals who showed signs of illness caused by trichinae during life. In general, the observations recorded by other investigators in the course of the recent surveys of over 5,500 human diaphragms also show a high incidence (14 percent) and a low intensity of infection. Practically none of the investigators who conducted the surveys were able to obtain from the medical history of the persons involved any conclusive evidence of clinical trichinosis during life.

The number of cases of clinical trichinosis in the United States actually recorded as such in the medical literature is very small when compared with the high incidence of infection with trichinae already discussed. In 1938 Sawitz (*13*) concluded from a study of the statistical data published by the United States Public Health Service and records available in medical journals that the total number of cases of clinical trichinosis ever recorded in the United States amounts to between 5,000 and 6,000. It cannot be properly concluded, however, that all cases of trichinosis that have occurred in this country since 1842, when these parasites were first found in the body of a person who had suffered rheumatic pains in the arms and legs, have found their way into medical statistics or into the medical literature (*15*).

Investigations on the incidence of trichinae in human beings in foreign countries, comparable to those made in the United States, are only fragmentary. The recent examination of 200 diaphragm samples from as many persons who died in England from various causes disclosed only two lightly infected ones, thus giving an incidence of 1 percent (*24*). Recently an examination of 420 diaphragms in Canada (*2*) revealed 7 that were infected with trichinae, an incidence of 1.6 percent.

In England up to 1940, the number of cases of clinical trichinosis and those involving the post mortem discovery of trichinae in human cadavers was well below 100 (*24*). Because of this the general opinion has prevailed that that country was singularly free from the disease. However, a serious epidemic of trichinosis came to light in England in December 1940, as previously noted, with an estimated number of at least 500 clinical cases and an undetermined number of nonclinical infections. It is quite evident, therefore, that as long as infected animals exist as a reservoir of the disease, the danger of its spreading to man is ever present.

Occurrence and Frequency of Trichinae in Swine in the United States

The first recorded discovery of trichinae in swine was made in the United States in 1866 by Leidy, who discovered the cysts while eating a slice of cooked pork in his home in Philadelphia (*7*).

In 1862, 2 years after the discovery of the transmission of trichinae to man as a result of the consumption of raw, infected pork, an epidemic of trichinosis, with the mortality of 16 percent, came to light in a small town in Germany. Two years later another and even more serious epidemic of this disease occurred in another small town in that country, with the result that pork began to acquire the stigma of being capable of producing a serious and painful human disease that had a strikingly high mortality. These and other epidemics of trichinosis in Europe were not without effect on the American meat industry, which by 1879 had developed a rather flourishing export trade to certain countries in Europe. By 1881 Italy, Germany, Austria, and France had promulgated sanitary regulations prohibiting the importation of pork from the United States because of the alleged danger of acquiring trichinosis from this meat.

It is not surprising, therefore, that under the Federal meat-inspection act of 1891 provision was made for the microscopic examination for trichinae of pork intended for export to foreign countries in order to surmount the sanitary barriers that had been set up against the importation of this commodity from the United States. This led to the systematic microscopic examination of samples of muscle tissue from millions of hogs intended for export, and the microscopists of the Bureau of Animal Industry engaged in this work determined that a small percentage of these animals were actually infected with trichinae. In a total of over 8 million hogs samples of which were examined microscopically from 1898 to 1906, nearly 1.5 percent were found to contain live trichinae, and in addition slightly over 1 percent were found to contain what were, presumably, trichinae in various stages of disintegration.

With the passage of a new meat-inspection act by Congress in 1906, microscopic inspection for trichinae of pork intended for export was discontinued, largely because this inspection was inherently imperfect. According to statements published by European meat-inspection experts, reinspection of samples of pork from this country certified as being free from trichinae in accordance with the results obtained by microscopic inspection here showed some of the pork to be infected. The incidence of trichinae in swine in this country from 1906 up to quite recently was unknown but was assumed to be the same as that brought to light by the systematic microscopic examinations of 1898-1906.

In 1933 the writer initiated an investigation to determine the current frequency of infection of swine with trichinae, using for this purpose a procedure that gives far more accurate results than the microscopic inspection previously used. The new procedure consists in digesting in artificial gastric juice in an incubator the diaphragms of hogs, selected at random, and determining the number of trichinae, if any, present in each diaphragm in relation to the quantity of meat digested. Since the diaphragm is known to be one of the preferred locations of trichinae, it is believed that the procedure outlined establishes the true incidence of these parasites in swine to a higher degree of probability than any other known method of examination.

Out of more than 13,000 diaphragms from as many farm-raised hogs shipped to the most important meat-slaughtering centers of the United States, only 126 (0.95 percent) were found to be infected with trichinae. Nearly two-thirds of these contained the parasites in exceedingly small numbers (only 1 to 5 larvae per 100 grams–about 3½ ounces–of meat), so small, in fact, that it is doubtful whether any method of inspection other than the one used would have resulted in their discovery except by sheer accident. Considering the fact that in microscopic inspection of pork for trichinae only 3 samples from each carcass, each sample about the size of an oat grain and certainly no larger than a small pea, are examined or can be examined satisfactorily from a practical standpoint, it is quite evident that the chances of detecting such light infections are exceedingly slight.

Data not previously published show that out of about 9,000 samples of pork from as many hogs originating on the Atlantic and Pacific seaboards and known to have been fed almost exclusively on untreated garbage, 554 (6.11 percent) were found to be infected. Not only was the incidence of infection in the garbage-fed hogs greater than that in the farm-raised hogs fed forage, grain, and other feeds, but the intensity of infection in the garbage-fed series also was much greater. Only something over one-third of the diaphragms from the garbage-fed-samples contained the very light infections that occurred in about two-thirds of the positive diaphragms of farm-raised hogs. In one series, including nearly 4,500 diaphragms from garbage-fed hogs in one of the Pacific Coast States, the incidence of infection was over 3.5 percent. In another series including over 2,500 diaphragms from as many hogs from one of the Atlantic Seaboard States, the incidence of infection was about 10.5 percent, while in about 2,000 diaphragms from hogs in another State on the Atlantic coast the incidence was nearly 6 percent. It is evident, therefore, that the average frequency of trichinae in garbage-fed hogs is more than 6 times that in farm-raised hogs. Pork from hogs fed garbage is, therefore, a far greater danger to human health than that from hogs raised on the farm and fed on forage, grain, and the usual supplements of tankage and minerals.

In the course of examinations to determine the incidence of trichinae in swine fed on different types of feeds, over 2,200 diaphragms were obtained from hogs known to have been fed cooked garbage only. Of these, only 11 (slightly less than 0.5 per cent) were found to be infected, the numbers of trichinae in the positive hogs being very small. It is evident, therefore, that the danger inherent in garbage as a feed for swine, from the standpoint of trichinosis, is the presence in it of pieces of raw pork or other meat containing trichinae. Cooking destroys nearly all of these parasites, as shown by the data just presented, and would destroy all of them if sufficient heat were applied.

The occurrence of trichinae in nearly 1 percent of farm-raised hogs affords conclusive evidence that the animals must have had access at one time or another to offal, garbage, kitchen scraps, or possibly other sources of trichinous meat. In the absence of such sources of infection, these pigs would not acquire trichinae unless, because of some dietary deficiency or other reason, they happened to eat infected rats or mice.

According to information published recently (*14*), trichinae are now exceedingly rare in swine in Germany, as shown by the fact that in 1936 samples of only 135 hogs were found to be infected out of nearly 19 million swine, samples of which were examined under the microscope as a regular routine. The indicated frequency is about 7 infected hogs in every million examined. In Poland, where pork is not microscopically inspected for trichinae, the incidence of these parasites in swine was reported in a German publication in 1941 to be about 70 times greater than in Germany (*14*). In Canada, where swine-husbandry practices are more nearly similar to these prevailing in the United States than are those in European countries, an examination of 995 diaphragms from as many garbage-fed swine from the Provinces of Quebec, Ontario, and Manitoba disclosed 2 that were infected, the incidence being, therefore, 0.2 percent (*1*). This low figure is not surprising since the Dominion laws require the sterilization by heat of all garbage fed to swine. In a previous investigation in Canada involving nearly 2,300 diaphragms the incidence of infection was 0.57 percent, very close to the figure derived from the data on the results of examinations in the United States of diaphragms of swine fed only cooked garbage.

Control of Trichinosis

Since there is no specific treatment for the removal of adult trichinae from the intestine or for the destruction of their larvae in the blood or muscles before or after their encystment, the major emphasis must be placed on prevention. Preventive measures must be directed against trichinosis in swine as well as in man because the successful control of the infection in pigs will result in a diminution in the number of human cases and might bring about its ultimate elimination from the list of human diseases. Actually, trichinosis in man is an easily preventable disease, since prevention consists merely in thoroughly cooking pork in all its forms. Its persistence despite repeated warnings of the danger inherent in raw pork is proof that warnings have not reached the public or that they have not been heeded by persons whose taste for raw pork in one form or another is such that they will eat it even in the face of the danger of acquiring a painful, serious, and possibly fatal illness.

Different countries have met the problem in different ways, the preventive measures adopted in any particular country being governed to a greater or less extent by the prevailing habits of the population with respect to the cooking and curing of pork and its products. Some countries have no trichinosis problem so far as is known, presumably because their populations do not eat raw pork in any form. Other countries, particularly on the continent of Europe, followed the leadership of Germany and long ago adopted as part of their meat-inspection procedure the plan of microscopic examination of samples of pork from all hogs slaughtered for human consumption, including those slaughtered on the farm for home consumption. In adopting this procedure, the meat-inspection authorities of the countries concerned recognized that they had to cope with the custom of eating pork in the raw state, a habit so deeply rooted in the general population that it could not, in their opinion, be eradicated by education. The countries that have practiced microscopic inspection, particularly Germany and Denmark, point with pride to the fact that, largely as a result of this, the incidence of trichinae in swine has declined steadily and that this decline has been reflected in a sharp diminution of trichinosis in man.

In the United States microscopic inspection for trichinae was resorted to, as previously noted, only in the case of pork intended for export to countries in Europe that made such inspection mandatory. The motives were economic rather than hygienic. At no time did American meat-inspection authorities give serious consideration to the adoption of microscopic inspection of pork for trichinae as part of the general procedure under Federal meat inspection. Investigations have shown that in numerous instances trichinous pork had been examined microscopically as many as 20 to 30 times before the parasites were found. Since it would be impracticable under any inspection scheme to make so many examinations, the unreliability of inspection for trichinae is quite obvious. Stiles (*23*) determined that out of 6,329 cases of trichinosis that occurred in Germany between 1881 and 1898, 2,042 (over 32 percent) could be traced to pork which had been inspected microscopically and passed as free from trichinae. This evidence shows that microscopic inspection is inherently imperfect and is fraught with the danger of giving persons who are fond of raw pork and its products a false sense of security, encouraging the consumption of raw pork and defeating in a measure the very purpose for which the inspection was intended.

It must be borne in mind that Federal meat inspection in this country is limited to plants that engage in interstate or foreign commerce. Slaughtering and meat-processing plants not engaged in interstate or foreign commerce do not come under the provision of the Meat Inspection Act and are therefore either without inspection or subject only to State or municipal inspection. Slaughtering done on the farm is exempt from inspection. Since only a few States and comparatively few municipalities have a rigid system of meat inspection, not all pork from hogs slaughtered in this country would be subjected to microscopic inspection even if such inspection were enforced in Government-inspected establishments. Actually, only about 60 percent of the hogs consumed in this country are slaughtered in Federally inspected establishments. It cannot be supposed that consumers would take the trouble in most instances to differentiate between pork inspected microscopically by Federal or other authorities and pork not so inspected. This situation would tend to nullify, at least in part, the good that might result from microscopic inspection of pork for trichinae. In addition, the cost of microscopic inspection by the Federal Government alone would involve an expenditure of about 10 million dollars annually (*17*), approximately twice the present outlay for all Federal meat inspection. In view of the fact that this investment of public funds cannot be expected to yield entirely satisfactory results, for the reasons already given, the drain on the Public Treasury that it would entail hardly appears to be warranted.

Following the publication of results of investigations showing that rabbits experimentally infected with trichinae gave clear-cut reactions to the injection into the skin of various test materials (antigens) prepared from trichina larvae, research work was undertaken by specialists in the Bureau of Animal Industry and elsewhere to determine the feasibility of detecting infection with trichinae in hogs prior to slaughter. Although several workers have recommended, at least by implication, the adoption of this or a similar biological test to weed out trichina-infected swine, the work reported by investigators of the Bureau of Animal Industry (*18, 19, 21, 22*) shows that the skin test, when applied to swine, is not sufficiently specific to warrant its use for the purposes indicated.

In the absence of any known practical method of inspection of hogs for trichinae, the regulations governing meat-inspection by the United States Department of Agriculture provide that no article of a kind prepared customarily to be eaten without cooking shall contain any muscle tissue of pork unless this meat has been subjected to a temperature sufficient to destroy all live trichinae, or to other treatment prescribed by the Chief of the Bureau of Animal Industry. The treatments prescribed for all meat food products containing pork muscle tissue that are prepared to be eaten without cooking are (1) heating, (2) special refrigeration, and (3) special processing. When heating is done, it is required that all meat food products of the kinds mentioned must be so heated that they will attain in all parts a temperature of not less than 137° F., this temperature having been determined by investigation to be lethal to trichinae (*12*). The required refrigeration involves the subjection of pork or of articles containing pork muscle tissue to a temperature of not less than 5° F. for a continuous period of not less than 20 days, or the subjection of the meat or articles to lower specified temperatures for shorter specified periods. Special curing methods in lieu of the required heating or refrigeration are designed to effect the destruction of trichinae by the action of curing ingredients, especially salt, by smoking at temperatures lower than 137° F. for definite periods, and by drying. The prescribed curing methods are known, as a result of numerous trials, to be effective in destroying the vitality of trichinae.

All the methods approved by the Bureau of Animal Industry as effective in destroying life in trichinae are based on extensive scientific research carried out in the laboratory and in meat-packing establishments and were subjected to repeated trials before they were adopted for official use. Under Federal meat inspection, therefore, the public is safeguarded against the danger of acquiring trichinosis from meat food products containing pork muscle tissue that are usually eaten without cooking. In preparing fresh pork and ordinary varieties of cured pork that have not been specially processed, under competent inspection, to destroy trichinae, the only safe rule to follow is to cook the pork until it is well done throughout.

In as much as data that have been presented in this article show that garbage-fed hogs have an average incidence of trichina infections more than six times that of farm-raised hogs and that cooking garbage renders it safe as a swine feed so far as trichinae are concerned, the control of garbage feeding by States and municipalities, through the enforcement of heat-sterilization requirements, or the voluntary adoption by feeders of the practice of sterilizing garbage by heat, would go a long way toward reducing the rather high incidence of trichinae in swine in the United States.

On the farm, three precautions would further reduce the incidence of swine trichinosis:

(1) Do not feed offal, kitchen scraps containing raw pork, or the contents of the slop barrel to swine;

(2) Do not throw dead rats and mice into the hog pens;

(3) Bury deeply in quicklime or burn the carcasses of hogs and other animals that die on the farm.

These steps, together with the control of garbage feeding indicated above, would eliminate to a large extent practically the only source of human trichinosis in this country.

Literature Cited

(1) CAMERON, THOMAS W.M. (1940). INVESTIGATIONS ON TRICHINOSIS IN CANADA. III. ON THE INCIDENCE OF TRICHINOSIS IN GARBAGE-FED HOGS. Canad. Jour. Res. Sect. D, Zool. Sci., 18: 83-85.

(2) EKBAUM, ELLA KUITUNEN (1941). THE INCIDENCE OF HUMAN TRICHINOSIS IN TORONTO. (Abstract of paper) Canad. Pub. Health Jour. 32: 78.

(3) HEMMERT-HALSWICK, ALFRED, and BUGGE, G. (1934). TRICHINEN UND TRICHINOSE. Ergeb. der Allg. Path. Mensch. u. Tiere 28: 313-392, illus.

(4) KERR, K.B., JACOBS, LEON, and CUVILLIER, EUGENIA (1941). STUDIES ON TRICHINOSIS. XIII. THE INCIDENCE OF HUMAN INFECTION WITH TRICHINAE AS INDICATED BY POST-MORTEM EXAMINATION OF 3,000 DIAPHRAGMS FROM WASHINGTON, D.C., AND 5 EASTERN SEABOARD CITIES. U.S. Pub. Health Serv., Pub. Health Rpts. 56: 836-855.

(5) LEE, J.E. STANLEY (1941). AN OUTBREAK OF TRICHINIASIS IN WOLVERHAMPTON AND DISTRICT. A CLINICAL ACCOUNT OF SEVEN CASES. Brit. Med. Jour. 4180: 237-240.

(6) LEIDY, JOSEPH (1848). [ENTOZOON IN THE SUPERFICIAL PART OF THE EXTENSOR MUSCLES OF THE THIGH OF THE HOG.] (Abstract) Acad. Nat. Sci. Phila. Proc. (1846-47) 3: 107-108.

(7) _____(1866). [REMARKS ON TRICHINA]. (Abstract) Acad. Nat. Sci. Phila. Proc. 18: 9.

(8) LEUCKART, RUDOLF (1876). DIE MENSCHLICHEN PARSITEN UND DIE VON IHNEN HERRUHRENDEN KRANKHEITEN: Bd. 2, 882 pp. Leipzig and Heidelberg.

(9) MATOFF, KONSTANTIN, and WAPZAROWA, MARA (1937). WIEVIEL JUNGTRICHINELLEN KANN EINE WEIBLICHE DARMTRICHINELLE GEBAREN. Ztschr. f. Infektionskrank., Parasitare Krank. u. Hyg. der Haustiere 51: 89-98.

(10) OWEN, RICHARD (1835). DESCRIPTION OF A MICROSCOPIC ONTOZOON INFESTING THE MUSCLES OF THE HUMAN BODY. [London] Zool. Soc. Trans. 1: 315-324, illus.

(11) QUEEN, FRANK R. (1931). THE PREVALENCE OF HUMAN INFECTION WITH TRICHINELLA SPIRALIS. (Abstract of paper) Jour. Parasitol. 18: 128.

(12) RANSOM, B.H. and SCHWARTZ, BENJAMIN (1919). EFFECTS OF HEAT ON TRICHINAE. Jour. Agr. Res. 17: 201-221.

(13) SAWITZ, WILLI (1938). PREVALENCE OF TRICHINOSIS IN THE UNITED STATES. U.S. Pub. Health Serv., Pub. Health Rpts. 53: 365-383, illus.

(14) SCHAAF, J. (1941). VORKOMMEN UND VERBREITUNG DER TRICHINOSE IM GENERALGOUVERNEMENT POLEN. Berlin. u. Munchen. Tierarztl. Wchnschr. Nr. 11: 131-133.

(15) SCHWARTZ, BENJAMIN (1929). TRICHINOSIS, A DISEASE CAUSED BY EATING RAW PORK. U.S. Dept. Agr. Leaflet 34, 8pp., illus.

(16) _____(1938). ANIMAL PARASITES TRANSMISSIBLE TO MAN. Sci. Monthly 47: 400-410.

(17) _____(1941). MEAT-INSPECTION ASPECTS OF TRICHINOSIS. Amer. Vet. Med. Assoc. Jour., 98: 459-461.

(18) _____and McINTOSH, ALLEN (1929). SKIN REACTIONS IN EXPERIMENTAL TRICHINOSIS IN PIG. (Abstract of paper) Jour. Parasitol. 16: 104-105.

(19) _____McINTOSH, ALLEN, and MITCHELL, W.C. (1930). NON-SPECIFIC SKIN REACTIONS IN PIGS TO THE INJECTION OF TRICHINA EXTRACTS. (Abstract of paper) Jour. Parasitol. 17: 114.

(20) SHELDON, J.H. (1941). AN OUTBREAK OF TRICHINIASIS IN WOLVERHAMPTON AND DISTRICT. Lancet [London] 1: 203-205.

(21) SPINDLER, L.A., and CROSS, S.X. (1939). INTRACUTANEOUS TESTS FOR THE DETECTION OF TRICHINA INFECTIONS EXPERIMENTALLY AND NATURALLY ACQUIRED BY SWINE. Helminthol. Soc. Wash. Proc. 6: 37-42.

(22) _____CROSS, S.X., and AVERY, J.L. (1941). RESULTS OF INTRACUTANEOS TESTS FOR THE DETECTION OF TRICHINA INFECTIONS IN SWINE. Helminthol. Soc. Wash. Proc. 8: 1-5.

(23) STILES, CHARLES WARDELL (1901). TRICHINOSIS IN GERMANY. U. S. Bur. Anim. Indus: Bul. 30, pp. 7-192.

(24) VAN SOMEREN, VERNON D. (1937). THE OCCURRENCE OF SUBCLINICAL TRICHINOSIS IN BRITAIN. RESULTS FROM 200 LONDON NECROPSIES. Brit. Med. Jour. 4014: 1162-1165.

Chapter 11

SALT TOLERANCE AND SALT POISONING OF SWINE

N.R. Ellis[1]

[1]*N.R. Ellis is Senior Chemist in Charge of General Nutrition Investigations. Animal Nutrition Division, Bureau of Animal Industry.*

There has been a good deal of discussion about whether certain cases of poisoning in swine, often fatal, were due to an excess of salt. The author reports the results of a careful investigation to clear up the whole question of how much salt swine can tolerate and what an excessive amount does to them.

Common salt is recognized as one of the chemical substances required in the diet of animals; hence it is good husbandry to include a supply in the rations of livestock. The quantitative requirements vary with the species. Those for swine are regarded as among the lowest. That excessive amounts may be harmful to the extent of being toxic is not at all surprising, since there are recognized limits beyond which various nutritive essentials become a burden, or even toxic, to the animal body. Much of the science of animal nutrition is built around the proper proportioning and balancing of the essential elements of the diet.

"Salt poisoning" is the term frequently used to characterize cerrtain forms of poisoning, often fatal, in swine, which are generally attributed to an excessive intake of sodium chloride. The true cause, particularly the conditions under which severe poisoning may result, remains obscure.

Various reports have listed a number of gross symptoms as characterizing the condition, including extreme nervousness, frothing at the mouth, convulsions, paralysis, diarrhoea, vomiting, loss of appetite, extreme thirst, blindness, and finally death. As evidence of the causative agent, case histories have frequently pointed to the consumption of large amounts of salt, especially in the form of brine, by hogs that for extended periods had not received salt as a regular part of their ration. Udal (*11*)[2] has pointed out that the immediate effect of excessive consumption of salt is inflammation of the mucous membrane of the stomach and marked redness and dryness of that of the mouth. The principal change evident on post mortem examination is gastroenteritis (inflammation of the stomach and intestines).

Results of Studies of Salt Requirements and Salt Tolerance of Swine

As a result of feeding investigations on the requirements of swine for salt, the need for small additions to the ration is well recognized. The generally recommended practice is to provide a mineral mixture containing salt in a self-feeder compartment, so that the pigs can satisfy their craving for minerals, or to mix small amounts with the concentrate feeds. The daily requirements are known to be small. Morrison (*7*) recommends not over ¼ pound of salt to 100 pounds of feed mixture. This would allow 5 to 6 grams (less than ¼ ounce) a day per 100 pounds of live weight; when this is added to the salt naturally contained in the average ration, the total would probably seldom exceed 10 grams (about 1/3 ounce).

That salt may be toxic to animals when consumed in large quantities has been recognized as entirely probable for a long time. The lethal, or fatal, dose for poultry has been fairly well established from the work of Mitchell, Card, and Carman (*6*) and others. Concerning the toxic quantity for swine, the results are conflicting. As will be, seen in the present review, the case against salt as the cause of poisoning is not clear-cut in spite of the frequent warnings found in textbooks and popular articles on swine feeding.

[2] Italic numbers in parentheses refer to Literature Cited.

Undoubtedly, gorging with salt has been at least a contributory if not the main factor in a certain number of deaths among swine. In his discussion of salt poisoning in livestock Udall (*11*) states that "swine have been poisoned by drinking brine and by eating garbage that had been pickled in brine." He quotes the toxic dose of salt for swine as ½ to 1 pound.

In reviewing his experiences with salt poisoning, Hofferd (*3*) observes that the most common effects of excessive salt intake over extended periods are inflammation of the kidneys and bladder and hardening of the liver. Acute poisoning was attributed to the consumption of brine. He states that diagnosis is often difficult because of varying symptoms. However, the temperature of affected animals generally remains about normal, and the animals usually show extreme nervousness and evidences of pain as a result of irritation of the kidneys and bladder. Among the instances of poisoning cited was one that occurred on a farm where a commercial mixed cattle feed containing much more salt than the hog feed in use was inadvertently placed in the hog feeders. In another instance a herd of pigs had been vaccinated with both virus and serum, and when a number of them sickened and became paralyzed the owner placed blocks of medicated salt in the pens. The pigs were observed to eat considerable amounts of the salt, and thereafter a number of the sick ones died. Removal of the salt blocks coincided with cessation of the deaths.

The consumption of salt in the form of brine is singled out by Hofferd and other writers as the chief factor in causing acute poisoning and sudden death of swine. Buffagni (2) has reported cases of poisoning in pigs due to a mixture of brine with the concentrate feed. A cow was reported as having been poisoned by 1 kilogram ($2^1/_5$ pounds) of salt administered as treatment for a condition diagnosed as indigestion.

Wautie (*13*), describing experimental work on salt and brine poisoning, tells that three pigs fed a brine solution that gave them 60 to 80 grams (2 to 3 ounces) of salt daily were severely affected by the tenth day. The symptoms consisted of stiffness of the legs, absence of reflex response, blindness, and constipation. An injection of calcium gluconate gave relief. Dry salt up to 250 grams (a little over half a pound) a day did not produce the extreme symptoms observed in the pigs given brine. He concluded that salt poisoning depends on the form in which the salt is taken (liquid or solid), the availability of water, the tolerance of the animal, and the type of food it is receiving. The poisoning from brine was thought to be due partly to the presence and action of nitrates, propylamine, and trimethylamine.

In recent years a number of workers have studied the salt tolerance of pigs in relation to their appetite for salt and to optimum and toxic levels. Amounts up to 80 grams (nearly 3 ounces) per animal per day increased the live-weight gains, and an intake of a gram per kilogram of live weight was not toxic, according to Vil'ner et al. (*12*). The ingestion of 100 grams (3½ ounces) a day over a 7-day period had no appreciable effect on the level of chloride in the blood in experiments reported by Marcq and Devuyst (*4*). Another conclusion that appears to be of special significance was that poisoning was difficult to cause experimentally except where secondary disorders were present. Tocher (*10*) concluded that pigs will not consume rations high in salt unless the salt is added gradually. He gave the optimum amount of salt with rations of mixed cereal, as approximately ½ ounce daily per 100 pounds of live weight.

In a study of the effect on swine of fish meals containing large amounts of salt, Rasenack (*8*) observed that pigs weighing 30 to 40 pounds showed signs of injury after consuming 15 grams (over ½ ounce) of salt daily. Serious injury and death did not results, however, until the level reached 75 or 100 grams daily (2½ to 3½ ounces). Another study on fish meal, by Mayrhofer (*5*), indicated that meals with as much as 9 percent of salt can be used without ill effects.

In view of the varying levels of sodium chloride naturally contained in swine rations and the disagreement in the recommendations on the optimum level, Sinclair (*9*) undertook some studies in which the salt additions were varied from none to 3 percent. The calculated daily total sodium chloride intake ranged from less than 0.1 gram in the basal grain ration to approximately 75 grams (2.7 ounces) in the ration with 3 percent of salt added. He estimated the daily sodium chloride requirement for a pig increasing in weight at the rate of 1 pound a day as 1.33 grams (about one-twentieth of an ounce). Apparently the sodium chloride contributed by tankage was sufficient to supply the needs of the pigs fed the grain-tankage diets used by Sinclair (*9*), since additions of salt to the diet did not increase the growth rates or efficiency of feed utilization of the pigs. From the standpoint of salt poisoning, no significant changes due to high salt intake were observed other than increase in water consumption and excessive urination. No changes were observed in the size or appearance of the kidneys, the water content of the muscle tissue, or the dressing percentage.

Interest in the often-repeated warning against salt poisoning led the Rowett Research Institute in Scotland to make a study of salt feeding (*1*). Pigs of 60 to 190 pounds live weight were fed a ration of cereal feeds, skim milk, cod-liver oil, and ground limestone, with different levels of sodium chloride. The pigs refused to eat a ration containing 4.7 percent of salt, and on a 3.3-percent salt level no apparent symptoms of ill health were noted. Further experiences, with pigs starved for 24 and 48 hours, led to the conclusion that pigs are unlikely to succumb to salt poisoning, because they refuse to eat salty feeds. The data on the optimum salt content of the ration for fattening pigs indicated a figure between 0.25 and 0.50 percent, which is in agreement with other published data.

Experiments at the Beltsville Research Centre

A somewhat different picture of the palatability of salt-containing rations, but with no change in the inability to produce toxic effects with any consistency, has been obtained in experiments with fattening pigs (results heretofore unpublished) at the Department of Agriculture Beltsville Research Centre, Beltsville, Md. In the first experiment, to a series of six diets, 0, 1, 2, 4, 8, and 12 percent, respectively, of salt was added. Two pigs were fed each diet. The average daily gains of the two pigs on the diet containing 2 percent of salt exceeded those of the other pigs. Increasing levels of salt resulted in decreased feed intake and retardation of gains. Nevertheless, the two pigs on the highest salt level ate sufficient feed to give them an intake of approximately half a pound of salt a day. One of the animals that received the diet with 8 percent of salt showed evidence of salt poisoning on the eighty-sixth day of the experiment. This pig, which had refused its feed for 2 days, when forced to move out of the shelter walked with a hesitant, nervous motion, frothed at the mouth, and champed its teeth. Two hours later, when it was driven with much difficulty to the scale house, the animal was quite evidently blind. Its weight was 160 pounds whereas

3 days previously it had weighed 187 pounds. A total of 1,770 cc. (1¾ quarts) of water was administered by mouth. Five days later when the animal was slaughtered it had fully recovered except for the blindness and weighed 197 pounds. It should be noted that while the development of blindness was attributed to the effects of the salt, the evidence is purely circumstantial. Microscopic examinations on the 12 hogs did not reveal any unusual changes attributable to salt ingestion.

In the second experiment, shotes were fed a ration containing only 0.1 percent of sodium chloride for 3- and 6-week periods and then given access to salt under various conditions, including free access to loose salt, salt mixed in different percentages in the dry feed, and free access to different brine concentrations. In no case were there any unusual effects that could be attributed in any way to salt poisoning. When the salt content of the diet was adjusted to 10 percent, the daily salt intake approximated 150 grams (5½ ounces) per 100 pounds of live weight. At a 15-percent level the feed intake was still not greatly depressed. The salt intake, however, increased in one case to approximately 180 grams (6.3 ounces) and in another to 225 grams (7.9 ounces) per 100 pounds live weight. Thus one animal weighing 218 pounds, after being fed 26 days on the high salt ration, was consistently consuming an average of 8.4 pounds of total ration, and 495 grams (1.1 pounds) of salt a day. A daily water consumption of 2.35 gallons at a period when water intake is normally low (December) was apparently sufficient to permit elimination of the salt without ill effects.

When brine solutions of 5- and 10-percent salt concentration were placed before two pigs that had received no added salt in the ration during a preliminary 3-week period, and no other water was furnished, relatively small amounts of the brine were consumed. One pig drank only 6 quarts of the 5-percent brine in 10 days, while the other consumed 5 quarts of 10-percent brine. Thus the daily salt intake was only a small fraction of that when salt was added to the ration. When two more pigs, after a preparatory period of 6 weeks without added salt were given access to the usual water supply in addition to the brine solutions, the brine consumption was of the same order as that of the pigs limited to brine only, namely, 4 to 5 quarts per 10-day period. The daily intake of salt in brine was thus only 40 to 60 grams (1.4 to 2.1 ounces) daily.

Two pigs were permitted free choice of dry salt without a preliminary salt-starvation period and four others (two in each group) after a 3-week and a 6-week salt-starvation period, respectively. In the first case (no salt-starvation period) the average daily salt intake amounted to only 5.5 grams. After a 3-week preliminary period the salt consumption averaged 12.7 grams a day, and after the 6-week period, 27 grams.

Two other animals were fed basal diets in which the salt content was increased at 7-day intervals by 4 percent each time. By the fifth week, the salt content was 20 percent, and it was maintained at this level for 4 weeks. The pigs grew normally for the first 4 weeks and maintained their weights with small fluctuations for the remaining 4 weeks. The water intake ranged between 6 and 8 gallons per pig per day during this time.

The 12 pigs used in these experiments were apparently in good health at the conclusion of the salt feeding. Several were changed back to the basal diet without salt additions for short periods previous to slaughter. When the pigs were slaughtered and examined, no unusual conditions were observed. Sodium chloride analyses of samples of lean tissue from the hams of the pigs that had received up to 20 percent of salt in their diets showed no significant difference from samples taken from hogs on ordinary diets.

Practical Conclusions

Considerable difficulty seems to attend the experimental production of salt poisoning by the direct use of salt. It is unfortunate that critical studies have not been made on the brine solutions that have reportedly caused toxic effects. Such studies might have disclosed the presence of other substances more definitely toxic than sodium chloride. Other secondary factors involving ailments difficult to diagnose are suggested in some of the reports.

Such practices as mixing salt with the mixed feeds in the slop barrel, dumping into the feeding troughs vats of old brine left over from the curing of meats, or adding to the feed batches of salt contaminated with unknown substances should be avoided in the feeding of swine. As already indicated, the salt requirements are so low and salt is so inexpensive that there is little justification for the use of waste products that might in one way or another be the cause of such cases of so-called salt poisoning as do occur.

The available evidence shows that there is considerable latitude in the tolerance of growing and fattening pigs for salt. In certain of the experiments cited, the pigs were induced to consume diets containing large amounts of salt, while in others the animals refused diets with even moderately high levels of salt. Undoubtedly the components of the diet and the previous feeding history play an important part. The low salt requirement of pigs was also emphasized in a number of instances. It would appear that the use of the animal-protein supplements and simple mineral mixtures containing moderate levels of salt such as are generally used by swine feeders in this country will seldom lead to salt hunger, much less to the setting up of conditions favourable to the intake of salt in unfavourable or toxic amounts.

Literature Cited

(1) BLISSETT, A.H. (1936). SOME RESULTS OF PIG FEEDING EXPERIMENTS OBTAINED AT THE DUTHIE EXPERIMENTAL STOCK FARM, ROWETT RESEARCH INSTITUTE. ABERDEEN. Pig Breeders' Ann. (1935-36) 15: 122-126.

(2) BUFFAGNI, VITTORIO (1935). AVVELENAMENTI DA CLORURO DI SODIO IN SUINI E BOVINI. Profilassi. 8: 53-54.

(3) HOFFERD, R.M. (1937). SALT POISONING IN SWINE. Norden News 11 (1): 6-7.

(4) MARCQ, J. and DEVUYST, A. (1935). INTOXICATION DE PORCS A L'ENGRAIS PAR LE SEL MARIN. Inst. Agron. et des Stas. de Rech. de Gembloux. Bul. 4: 316-324.

(5) MAYRHOFER, J. (1931). BEITRAG ZUR FRAGE DER VERFUTTERUNG SALZHALTIGER FISCHMEHLE. Fortschr. der Landw. 7: 230-231.

(6) MITCHELL, H.H., RCARD, L.E., and CARMAN, G.G. (1926). THE TOXICITY OF SALT FOR CHICKENS. Ill. Agr. Expt. Sta. Bul. 279, pp. 135-156. illus.

(7) MORRISON, FRANK BARRON (1936). FEEDS AND FEEDING. A HANDBOOK FOR THE STUDENT AND STOCKMAN. Ed. 20, unabridged, 1050 pp., illus. Ithaca, N.Y.

(8) RASENACK, OTTO (1925). UNTERSUCHUGEN UBER DIE WIRKUNG STARK KOCHSALZHALTIGEN FISCHMEHLS AUF SOHWEINE. Arch. f. Wiss. u. Prakt. Tierheilk. 52: 297-315.

(9) SINCLAIR, R.D. (1939). THE SALT REQUIREMENT OF GROWING PIGS. Sci. Agr. 20: 109-119, illus.

(10) TOCHER, J.F. (1935). THE PROPORTIONS OF CERTAIN POISONOUS SUBSTANCES IN FEEDING, STUFFS AND THEIR EFFECT ON LIVESTOCK. Vet. Rec. 15: [447]-480.

(11) UDALL, D.H. (1939). THE PRACTICE OF VETERINARY MEDICINE. Ed. 3, rev., 672 pp., illus. Ithaca, N. Y.

(12) VIL'NER, A., KRASOVSKY, I., and TSELIKE, B. (1936). [SODIUM CHLORIDE IN PIG FATTENING.] Svinovodstvo Nos. 9 and 10. [In Russian. Abstract in Nutr. Abs. and Rev. 7: 778. 1938.]

(13) WAUTIE, A. (1935). CONTRIBUTION A L'ETUDE DES ACCIDENTS CAUSES PAR LE SEL ET LA SAUMURE CHEZ LE PORC. Ann. de Med. Vet. 80: 253-261.

Chapter 12

NUTRITIONAL DISEASES OF SWINE

Louis L. Madsen[1]

[1] *Louis L. Madsen is Nutritionist, Animal Nutrition Division, Bureau of Animal Industry.*

The symptoms, causes, and prevention of the mineral and vitamin deficiencies that affect swine–often with serious consequences for the producer–are discussed in this article, which also includes the results of recent experiments with some of the little-known B vitamins.

The control of nutritional diseases among swine is one of the first essentials in successful pork production. The importance of adequate nutrition is further emphasized by the fact that the cost of feed alone, including pasture, is estimated as making up 65 to 85 percent of the total cost of producing hogs for market. Swine are able to convert a larger proportion of their feed into edible meat and fat than any other farm animal, but errors in diet which slow their growth or lead to poor utilization of feed or the development of nutritional diseases can result in heavy death losses and otherwise seriously interfere with the economical production of pork.

Many nutritional diseases of swine can be readily controlled if feed requirements are understood and the required nutrients are provided. Early recognition of deficiency symptoms and prompt application of curative or preventive measures will frequently prevent heavy losses. A knowledge of the nutritive value of feeds is very helpful in this respect.

Swine are raised under a wide variety of conditions and are fed many kinds of feed. Concentrated feeds make up the bulk of most ordinary rations, but some bulky feeds, such as good pasture plants or a limited amount of well-cured roughage (particularly alfalfa), have proved to be of value as sources of essential nutrients. Pigs fed in the dry lot and especially in floored pens depend entirely on their daily allowance of feed to meet their requirements. Such animals are particularly likely to suffer from nutritional diseases unless their ration is carefully selected.

Since this article deals primarily with the nutritional diseases of swine, for additional information on the nutritive requirements of swine and practices in swine feeding the reader is referred to articles in the 1939 Yearbook of Agriculture (*7, 31*).[2]

The Mineral-Deficiency Diseases of Swine

Calcium and Phosphorous Deficiency and the Interrelationship of Vitamin D

Calcium deficiency is more likely to occur in swine than a deficiency of phosphorus because swine are often fed rations made up largely of grains or grain by–products, together with some protein-rich concentrates, and these feeds are usually good sources of phosphorus but low in calcium. Vitamin D is closely related to the metabolism of calcium and phosphorus and is therefore considered with the deficiency diseases involving these two minerals.

Rickets

Rickets, a disease of young animals, occurring before the bones cease growing in length, is most often seen in winter and early spring when pigs are kept housed because of inclement weather, but it may occur at any time of the year if the animals are improperly fed and not allowed free access to direct sunlight.

The symptoms of rickets in swine (22) are similar to those in other young animals. Affected animals frequently have a poor appetite and a generally unthrifty appearance, soft, fragile bones,

---

[2] Italic numbers in parentheses refer to Literature Cited.

and usually lameness, especially in the advanced stages of the disease. The degree of bone and joint involvement varies; there may be merely a slight stiffness and stilted movements, or the animals may be able only to crawl on their knees; or they may lie on one side, unwilling or unable to get up. The front and hind legs may become bowed, and the joints are frequently enlarged. The pasterns in some pigs become abnormally straight and thickened, while in others they sag until the pigs almost walk on their dewclaws. In standing, the front and hind feet are often brought very close together. The back is usually abnormally arched.

In advanced cases of vitamin D deficiency, blood-serum calcium is usually lowered from a normal value of 10 to 12 milligrams per 100 milliliters to 6 milligrams or less. Blood phosphorus also may be low. At the lower levels of blood calcium, the animals may go into tetanic convulsions, frequently referred to as fits, and sometimes die in convulsions.

Symptoms appear earlier and their onset is somewhat more gradual in young weanling pigs than in older animals. Fattening pigs may "go off their feet" rather suddenly. Such animals usually lose appetite quickly, appear sick, and may have marked incoordination of movement or suffer from partial or complete paralysis. Broken or dislocated leg and pelvic bones or fractured vertebrae resulting in pressure on the nerves and spinal cord may be the cause of these symptoms in some cases. The death rate from rickets is not usually very high, but animals suffering from the disease may succumb to pneumonia or other communicable diseases to which they are predisposed by their weakened condition.

Cause, Prevention, and Treatment

Rickets is usually due to an inadequate intake of calcium or phosphorus or both, or to a faulty proportion of these minerals in the diet, together with a deficiency of vitamin D. A deficiency of vitamin D or of this vitamin and calcium is the chief cause of rickets in swine. Pigs fed indoors on a ration made up largely of cereal grains, without access to palatable sun-cured roughage, direct sunlight, or other source of vitamin D, are therefore very likely to develop this deficiency disease.

An adequate intake of vitamin D cannot compensate for faulty mineral nutrition. The quantitative requirement for vitamin D is lowest, however, when the ratio of calcium to phosphorus lies within the range of 1:1 or; 2:1 (2). Too much calcium in the ration interferes with the utilization of phosphorus. An excess in the diet of other minerals, such as salts of iron, magnesium, beryllium, manganese, strontium, thallium, and aluminium, may also interfere with phosphorus assimilation.

Rickets can be readily prevented or cured in the early stages by correcting the diet. Young pigs that have access to direct sunshine store up considerable amounts of vitamin D. It is not safe, however, to depend entirely on stored vitamin D during long feeding periods in confinement unless the pigs are fed in outdoor lots so that direct sunshine is available. When the body stores of this vitamin are largely depleted, rickets will develop. Johnson and Palmer (20) found that coloured pigs, when allowed access to fall sunshine before being confined for the winter, stored sufficient vitamin D to protect them from rickets for about 4 to 8 weeks, while white pigs under comparable conditions were protected about twice as long.

The most economical source of vitamin D is direct sunshine, but thus may be inadequate in northern latitudes during the winter. High-grade sun-cured legume hay, particularly alfalfa, is a very good source of vitamin D as well as of calcium. Alfalfa of good quality may be fed either free choice in racks or chopped or ground and added to the grain ration at the rate of 5 to 10 percent for fattening pigs and 10 to15 percent for sows and boars. Artificially dehydrated alfalfa meal is lower in vitamin D than meal made from sun-cured hay. Other hays, such as soybean, lespedeza, sweetclover, red clover, etc., may be used in place of alfalfa, although they are not usually as palatable. When a good grade of hay is not available for winter feeding and available sunshine is limited, vitamin D may be furnished by such supplements as fish oils, fortified oils, and such irradiated products as yeast and activated sterols of animal origin.

Insuring an adequate calcium and phosphorus intake is as important as supplying vitamin D. Many feeds, including buttermilk, skim milk, tankage, fish meal, and meat scraps, are rich in both calcium and phosphorus. Legume pasture and hay furnish an abundance of calcium, while wheat bran and the protein-rich meals such as linseed, cottonseed, and soybean are rich in phosphorus but low in calcium.

The choice of a mineral supplement, if any is needed, depends on the mineral content of the grain ration. Sources of calcium and phosphorus are often fed with common salt. Other essential minerals such as iodine, iron, and copper may be included in such a mixture when necessary. Some suggested mineral mixtures that can be very economically mixed on the farm according to the individual needs of pigs are given in Table 1. These mixtures may be fed free choice or added to the ration at the rate of 1 to 1½ pounds to each 100 pounds of grain mixture. Additional salt may be given free choice.

Table 1: Suggested Mineral Mixtures for Hogs

Mixture no.	*Mineral supplement needed*	*Suggested Mixture*		
		Ground Limestone	*Steamed bonemeal*	*Common salt*
		Pounds	Pounds	Pounds
1.	Very high calcium	75	-	25
2.	Very high calcium; medium phosphorous	50	25	25
3.	High calcium; high phosphorous	33⅓	33⅓	33⅓
4.	High calcium, very high phosphorous	-	75	25

Mineral supplement No.1 should be used when the ration is low in calcium only. Phosphorus in this case must be supplied by the rest of the ration of whole grains, grain byproducts, and protein-rich concentrates. As previously explained, excessive calcium feeding should be avoided. Mineral supplements No. 2 and No. 3 furnish large amounts of calcium and supply phosphorus in addition. Mixture No.3 is probably the most widely recommended mineral supplement and has been fed with success to swine of all ages as well as to other farm animals. Mineral supplements Nos. 2 and 3 are appropriate for rations that supply less phosphorus and may also be used successfully in the case of young breeding animals with which the total grain allowance is somewhat restricted to avoid excessive fattening. No. 4 furnishes calcium and more phosphorus than No. 2 or No. 3, but this is not often essential when ordinary well-balanced swine rations are fed. Bonemeal is usually more expensive as a source of calcium than a good grade of limestone or oystershell. Defluorinated rock phosphate prepared for animal feeding may also be used as a source of calcium and phosphorus.

Calcium Deficiency in Brood Sows

Breeding swine, particularly pregnant or lactating sows, develop serious symptoms if their ration is deficient in calcium. This deficiency is most common in swine fed in floored pens, without access to pasture, on a ration consisting largely of cereal grains without an appropriate mineral mixture. In a study of the effects of calcium deficiency on the general appearance and reproductive performance of sows and gilts, Evans (*8*) describes this condition as follows:

*** the main manifestations of calcium deficiency–as typified by all the pigs in the group-were:

(1) Rough scaly skins, dirty in appearance.
(2) The pigs were periodically "off their feet" with their legs bending inwards, and developed what appeared to be characteristic signs of rickets.
(3) The sows often refused their feed towards parturition, this indicating nutritive disturbances.
(4) They had great difficulty in farrowing and could not stand on their feet for two or three days afterwards.
(5) No signs of milk could be seen before or after farrowing, and their udder was very flabby especially in comparison with the normal sows.
(6) Very few pigs survived at weaning time and even the few left made very poor live weight gains. It should be observed, however, that the sows themselves when they farrowed appeared to be in good condition.

Hogan (*12*) in studying the calcium requirement of brood sows found that their rations should contain not less than 0.4 percent of calcium. Sufficient calcium will usually be furnished if 1 to 1½ pounds of mineral mixture No. 1 (Table 1) is added to the ordinary ration made up largely of cereal grains.

Good pasture and legume forage should be included in the ration of the brood sow whenever possible. Well-cured legume hay, particularly alfalfa, may be fed in a rack or ground and added to the grain mixture at the rate of 10 to 15 percent. When the ration of the sow contains such feeds as fish meal, tankage, buttermilk, and skim milk in liberal quantities, the intake of calcium and phosphorus is usually adequate, and it is unnecessary to supply these minerals in a special supplement.

Phosphorus Deficiency

As already noted, phosphorus is less likely to be deficient in ordinary swine rations than calcium (the reverse of the situation with cattle). When swine are grazed on pasture or on cultivated root crops with little or no grain and no protein-rich or phosphorus-rich mineral supplement, however, phosphorus deficiency may develop. Aubel, Hughes, and Leinhardt (*1*) fed swine on low phosphorus rations and reported the following symptoms:

* * * (1) A loss of appetite, (2) a poor utilization of feed and storage of energy, (3) a failure to make normal growth and to develop bone and muscle normally, (4) a lowering of inorganic phosphorus in the blood, and (5) a marked increase in thirst and a corresponding excretion of urine.

The increased water intake and excessive urine output were associated with enlarged kidneys, which were pale in colour.[3]

Under the conditions of the experiment, the phosphorus intake was adequate when the ration contained at least 0.27 to 0.3 percent of phosphorus.

Ordinary feeds that are good sources of phosphorus for swine are wheat bran, wheat middlings, and especially the protein-rich concentrates such as tankage, fish meal, and soybean, linseed, cotton-seed, and peanut meals. Dairy byproducts, such as skim milk and buttermilk, are good sources of phosphorus as well as of calcium. When phosphorus-rich feeds are used in the ration, it may not be necessary to supply additional quantities of phosphorus. In cases where additional phosphorus is needed, mineral mixtures Nos. 2, 3, or 4 (Table 1) may be offered the pigs in a self-feeder. Too much calcium in the ration will adversely affect the utilization of phosphorus.

Nutritional Anemia of Suckling Pigs

Nutritional anemia is one of the principal causes of unthriftiness and death among young swine. It is particularly prevalent in figs farrowed in late fall, winter, and early spring which, because of

---

[3] On histological examination these "large white kidneys" showed "chronic diffuse nephritis of the parenchymatous type and presented widened glomerular spaces around the glomerular tufts and also widely distended uriniferous tubules with flattened epithelial cells. A granular debris was present in some of the tubules.

inclement weather or for other reasons, are kept confined to floored pens without access to soil or vegetation. The condition usually appears in pigs 1 to 6 weeks of age, with a somewhat higher incidence about the third week of life. Affected pigs show paleness of the skin and the mucous membranes, lack of vigour, sluggishness, failure to gain normally in weight, and unusual fatigue and laboured breathing (thumps) on the slightest exertion. Young pigs may be severely anemic and yet appear fairly well developed and fat. Some lie suddenly; others linger for several weeks, lose condition, and become emaciated. Post mortem examination reveals watery blood, excessive fluid in body cavities, grayish-yellow, mottled liver, and marked paleness of the muscles, lungs, and kidneys. Pneumonia and digestive disturbances may also occur. Swine that have recovered from anemia frequently show scattered areas of fibrosis–formation of fibrous tissue-in the liver, due presumably to a healing and replacement process following damage during the anemia.

The milk of all animals is extremely poor in iron and copper, and since young swine are born with a limited store of these minerals, a regular supply is needed shortly after birth to meet the needs of increased blood formation and rapid growth. Soil and forage normally supply sufficient quantities of iron and copper, but newborn pigs kept in pens with surfaced floors or in paved lots have no opportunity to get these minerals. Anemia may also be caused by intestinal parasitism or may accompany severe disorders such as necrotic enteritis, but in these cases factors other than primary iron and copper deficiency are involved.

Several methods have proved successful in the control of anemia. Putting the sow and pigs out to pasture as soon as the weather and other conditions are satisfactory is a good way to prevent anemia. A few shovelfuls of sod or soil taken from areas not traversed by swine (to limit parasitic infestation) placed in the pen or lot may also provide ample protection, but it may be better to enrich the soil with iron and copper salts. Willman, McCay, and Morrison (*29*) were successful in preventing anemia in confined suckling pigs by treating them with a saturated solution of dried ferrous sulphate (copperas, 1 pound per quart of water, dissolved as completely as possible with hot water in the following ways:

(1) Drenching the pigs once a week until they are 4 or preferably 6 weeks old.

(2) Drenching them twice a week until they are 4 weeks old.

(3) Swabbing the udder of the sow once daily until the pigs are 6 weeks old.

One-third of a teaspoonful of the solution should be the maximum dose for pigs under 1 week of age. This dosage may be increased until the pigs are receiving 1 teaspoonful when they are about 3 or 4 weeks old. Drenching or swabbing, preferably the latter which is usually the most convenient method of controlling anemia, should be started when the pigs are 3 or 4 days old. It has been observed that too large doses of the iron solution given as a drench to young pigs will cause scours and occasionally vomiting. Treatment may be discontinued whenever the pigs are turned out to pasture. Pigs older than 6 weeks usually are eating enough supplementary feeds to prevent anemia. Extra iron need not be provided in salt mixtures for adult swine except in areas where the soil is deficient in this mineral.

Iodine Deficiency and the Birth of Weak Pigs

A deficiency of iodine in the ration of pregnant sows leads to the birth of weak off-spring. The young pigs may be still born

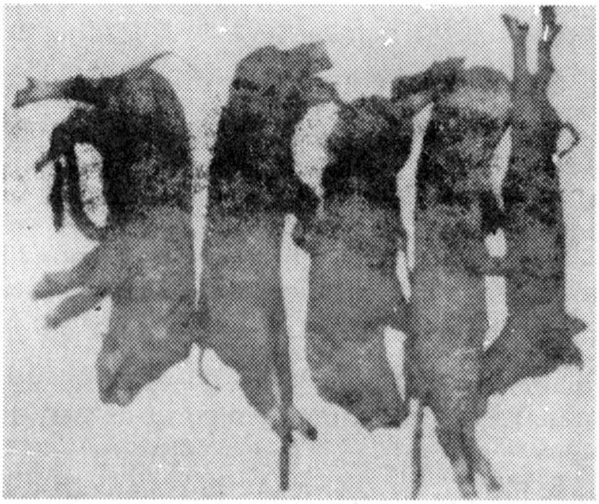

Fig. 1: A litter of hairless; pigs still born. The sow that farrowed them received too little iodine. (Courtesy of J.W. Kalkus, Western Washington Experiment Station).

(Fig. 1), or they may be born alive and dies shortly afterward. (*28*). The symptoms add prevention of this disease in swine and other farm animals are discussed in the article on Nutritional Diseases of Farm Animals.

Manganese Deficiency and Lameness in Pigs

Miller and co-workers (*24*) describe a lameness in pigs fed rations consisting of yellow corn, tankage, soybean meal, ground alfalfa, and salt. The condition is manifested by stiffness, enlarged hock joints, and crooked legs, as in rickets, but adding calcium and phosphorus or various sources of vitamin D is ineffective in treatment. In initial experiments, manganese sulphate added to the ration at the rate of 50 to 60 parts of manganese per million was effective in preventing the lameness but not in curing it once it was established. Wheat and oats are usually higher in manganese than corn.

Toxic Minerals

Fluorine and Selenium Poisoning

Fluorine and selenium poisoning of swine and other livestock is discussed in the article on Nutritional Diseases of Farm Animals. Kick, Bethke, and Edgington (*21*) found that pig rations containing 0.03 percent or more of fluorine derived either from rock phosphate or sodium fluoride were harmful.

Symptoms of fluorine poisoning in swine include slow growth, low feed consumption, stiffness, marked changes in the bones and teeth (Fig. 2), increased thirst, and kidney injury. The bones become thicker than normal, break more easily, and are rough, white, and lusterless. The mandibles (jawbones) are also enlarged and rough.

Swine suffering from the toxic effects of fluorine may improve considerably if the source of fluorine is eliminated from the ration, but they may be permanently injured to some extent.

Moxon (*25*) states that hogs seem to be even more susceptible than cattle and horses to selenium poisoning.

The Vitamin-Deficiency Diseases of Swine

Vitamin A Deficiency

Vitamin A deficiency occurs most commonly in swine fed in dry lots on rations of grain other than yellow corn, without access to

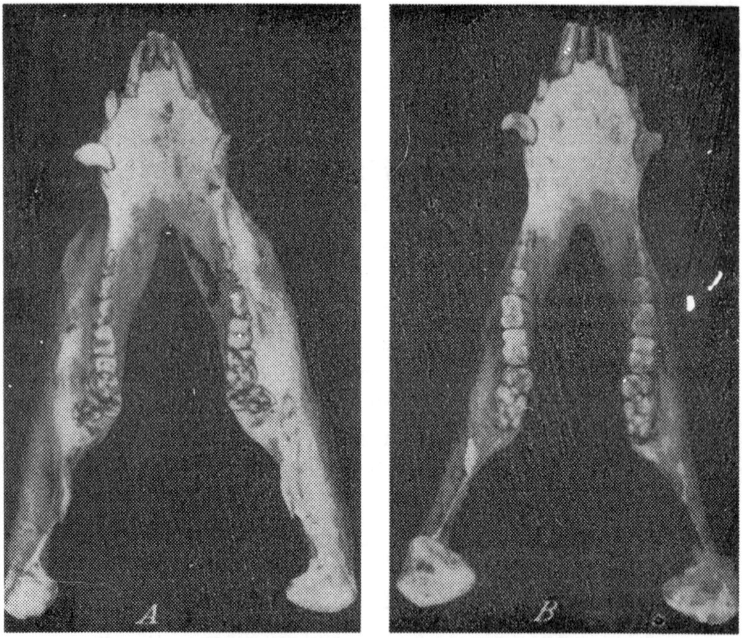

Fig. 2: "A" Thickened jawbone, the result of the consumption of too much fluoriue in raw rock phosphate. "B" A normal jaw, shown for comparison. (Courtesy R.M. Bethke, Ohio Agricultural Experiment Station).

green feed, well-cured forage, or other sources of carotene or vitamin A.

One of the earliest indications of the deficiency is night blindness, although Guilbert, Miller, and Hughes (*10*) found that in experimental vitamin A deficiency of swine some of the animals developed partial posterior paralysis before defective night vision had been demonstrated. Hostetler, Foster, and Halverson (*13*) found that pigs suffering from advanced vitamin A deficiency would easily become excited and fall over on one side in a spasm or convulsion, roll their eyes, struggling a little or lying with legs extended, squeal as if in pain, and give evidence of laboured breathing. The animals also had a watery discharge from the eyes and were partly or completely blind. Other symptoms are loss of appetite, diarrhoea, unthrifty appearance, staggering gait, and in the later stages complete incoordination of the hind limbs due to degeneration of the nerve and spinal cord. Gilts or sows usually show considerable irregularity in breeding behaviour. Some fail to breed entirely, while in others, according to Hughes, Aubel, and Lienhardt (*19*), the heat periods are more frequent than normal and of longer duration. They state:

> * * * The vulva of some of the gilts in the later stages of the disorder remained swollen as though in continuous cestrum. * * * The ovaries of these sows on examination showed the unusual condition of containing at the same time, ripe Graffian follicles, freshly ruptured follicles, and both new and old *corpora lutea*.

If a sow moderately deficient in vitamin A is bred, it may abort, or a resorption of the fetus may take place. In some cases the young may be born at the regular term but may be either dead or so weak that they die shortly after birth. In such cases the sow frequently fails to lactate normally. Hale (*11*) has made a series of interesting observations on embryonic injury to swine due to maternal vitamin A deficiency previous to and during the early period of gestation. He found various eye defects and abnormalities, including absence of eyes. There were various developmental defects, such as accessory ears, subcutáneous cysts, harelip, cleft palate, faulty kidney development, and malformed hind legs. (Fig. 3).

The value of green pasture or soiling crops (rape, soybeans, field peas, alone or in combination with cereal grains, etc). for sows and young growing swine cannot be overemphasized. On these feeds the young feeder pigs or breeding animals store up a considerable amount of vitamin A in their bodies, and these stores are utilized to good advantage later during periods of dry-lot fattening or in winter, when the supply of carotene-rich feeds is limited.

Well-cured, green, leafy legume hay, particularly alfalfa, is an excellent source of carotene and prevents acute vitamin A deficiency among swine in dry lots. If the hay is of good quality, a sufficient amount may be eaten if fed in racks; otherwise, 5 to 10 percent of alfalfa meal should be added to the gram ration of young fattening swine or 10 to 15 percent to the ration of breeding animals. When yellow corn is the principal grain fed, it can usually be depended on to furnish enough vitamin A for fattening animals, but there is still some question whether the amount needed for reproduction will be sufficient when furnished by yellow corn only. If a good grade of

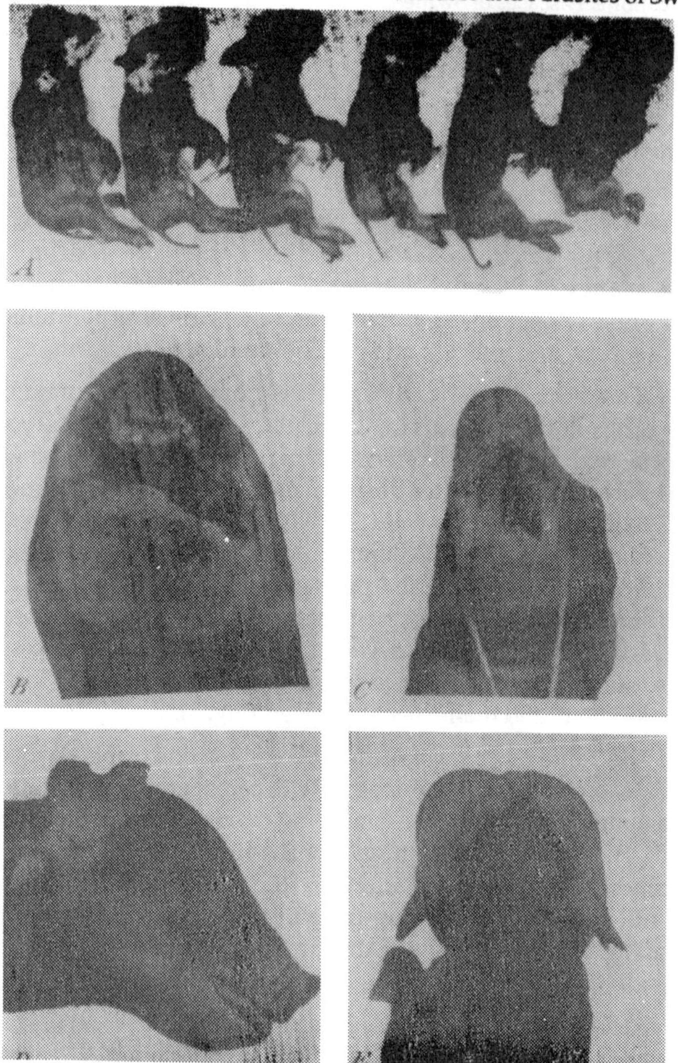

Fig. 3: Pigs born to sows that have been fed rations deficient in vitamin A may have various developmental abnormalities, are usually weak at birth, and often die. "A" A portion of a litter of 10 pigs all born without eyeballs. The pig on the left has a cystic enlargement on the head. "B" A pig with a double cleft lip. "C" A pig with a cleft palate. "D" and "E" show an eyeless pig with extra earlike growths. (Courtesy of Fred Hale, Texas Agricultural Experiment Station).

hay or alfalfa meal is not available, vitamin A may be furnished by cod-liver oil or some other fish oils. Other feeds rich in carotene are yellow sweet-potatoes and yellow carrots. Swine suffering from vitamin A deficiency will usually respond very quickly when the vitamin is supplied in adequate amounts, but animals with advanced symptoms such as marked muscular incoordination or blindness seldom recover completely.

Thiamin (Vitamin B_1) Deficiency

Symptoms of thiamin deficiency have recently been produced in swine by feeding experimental rations, but no direct evidence is available to indicate that pigs given ordinary feeds suffer from a deficiency. It is recognized, however, that the requirement for thiamin is very high for reproduction and lactation, though little attention has been given to this problem in the case of swine.

Hughes (*14, 15*) lists decrease in appetite with a tendency towards leg weakness, a lowering of body temperature, decreased respiratory rate, and, on autopsy, flabby heart with some changes in the digestive tract as characteristic symptoms in pigs on diets deficient in one or more vitamins of the B complex. Van Etten, Ellis, and Madsen (*27*) produced thiamin-deficiency symptoms by feeding nursling pigs diets treated with sodium sulphite and sulphur dioxide to destroy the vitamin. They found that after several weeks on the diet the young pigs started to refuse food, vomited occasionally, became emaciated, and had a marked lowering of the body temperature (Fig. 4). Death usually occurred within 5 weeks unless thiamin was added to the diet. On autopsy, a flabby heart and liver damage were often found. Some individuals have increased amounts of fluid in the body cavities and also pathological changes in the intestine. Histological (cell) changes were reported in the heart and liver. Electrocardiographic studies recently made in the Animal Nutrition Division, Bureau of Animal Industry, revealed a lowered heart rate and abnormalities of conduction in the heartbeat in thiamin deficiency.

Thiamin deficiency probably never occurs if the diet contains a liberal amount of whole cereal grains or if the animals have access to pasture or well-cured legume forage. Other feeds rich in thiamin are mill by-products (such as wheat bran), yeast, and legume seeds, such as beans, peas, and peanuts. Increasing the fat in a thiamin-deficient ration lowers the requirement.

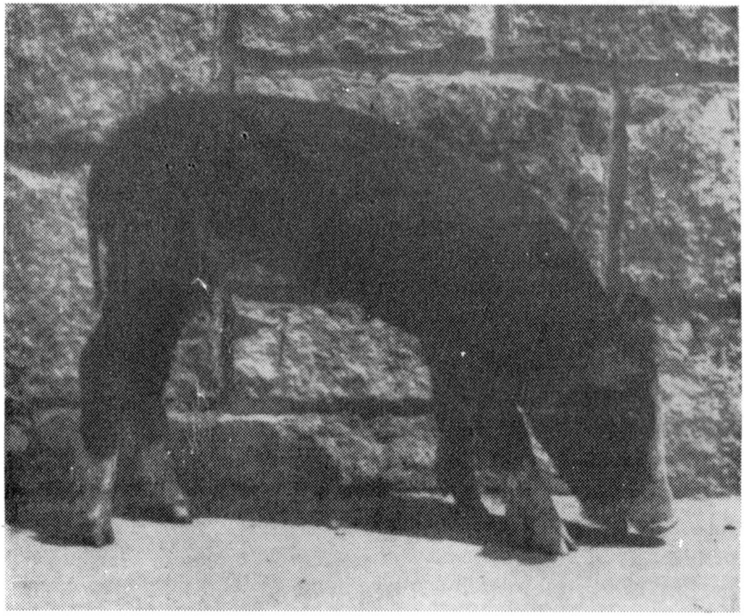

Fig. 4: This pig is showing the effects of thiamin (vitamin B_1) deficiency. The main symptoms are lack of appetite, emaciation, lowered body temperature, and slow heart rate.

Riboflavin Deficiency

Riboflavin deficiency has been produced experimentally by Hughes (*15*) by feeding a diet low in this factor. He describes the symptoms as slow growth, frequent scours, and walking with difficulty owing to a crippled condition of the legs. Feeding a source of flavin slightly improved the growth and well-being of the pigs, but no improvement was noted in their walking ability. Work in the Bureau of Animal Industry confirmed the fact that riboflavin is essential to swine. Nursling pigs fed a riboflavin-deficient diet failed to gro·v normal, vomited frequently, had severe diarrhoea, developed a rough skin and hair coat, had considerable secretion about the eyes, developed a peculiar gait, became very sick, and died (Fig. 5).

Hughes (*16*) reports that the minimum daily requirement of riboflavin for young growing swine is between 1 and 3 milligrams per 100 pounds of live weight. The value of dairy byproducts such

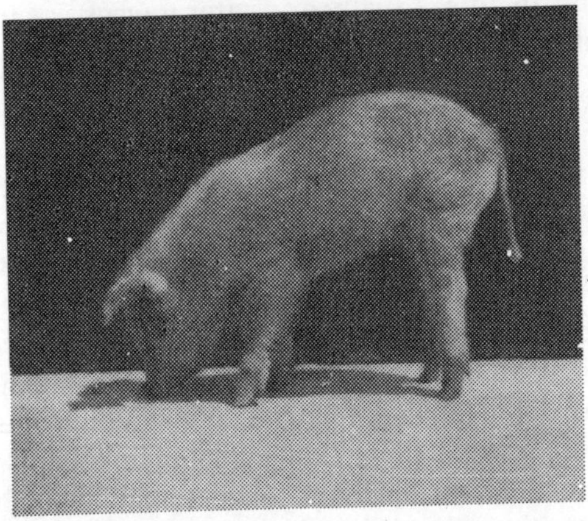

Fig. 5: Nursling pigs develop riboflavin deficiency within a very short time when given a diet low in this factor. Note poor condition, rough hair coat, and peculiar straight posture of hind legs of this pig.

as skim milk, buttermilk, and whey in swine feeding is probably partly due to their high riboflavin content. Yellow corn, an important swine food, is a fair source of riboflavin. Wheat and barley are lower in this vitamin.

Nicotinic Acid Deficiency and Necrotic Enteritis in Swine

When nicotinic acid therapy for blacktongue in dogs was announced in the United States, Chick and associates (3) in England had two young pigs that had developed a characteristic dietary disease from having been maintained on a Goldberger (pellagra-producing) corn diet. The principal symptoms were severe diarrhoea, refusing food, dirty-yellow skin, severe scabby dermatitis (skin inflammation), loss of hair, and a muscular difficulty in the use of the hind legs. Two intra muscular injections of 100 milligrams of nicotinic acid in one pig and three injections in the other at 3-day intervals, followed by a daily allowance of 60 milligrams in the food, produced a striking effect: The appetite returned within 24 hrs of the first injection, the diarrhoea abated and they began to increase in weight * * *. The scabs on the skin began to be detached after 1 week, leaving clean, healthy skin. At the same time, the colour of the animals improved gradually and after 6 weeks of treatment was that of healthy pigs.

At the time of this report, about 2 years' work at the Michigan station, started by Madsen and continued by Davis, was reported briefly by Gardner (9). This preliminary note pointed out that in certain feeding experiments swine developed intestinal disorders resembling necrotic enteritis and that supplementary feeds, such as raw liver, brought about remarkable recovery from the disease. Barley also had a preventive and curative influence. In some cases nicotinic acid was just as beneficial as liver. The Michigan work, later published in detail (5), suggests that necrotic enteritis is a secondary complication caused by intestinal invasion by organisms following nicotinic acid deficiency in the pig. It was pointed out, however, that necrotic enteritis probably involved additional dietary factors.

Common swine feeds, such as corn, milk, and milk byproducts and soybean and linseed meals, are relatively low in nicotinic acid. Peanut meal, however, is reported to be high in this factor. Barley is usually higher in nicotinic acid than corn, while wheat and oats have intermediate amounts.

In the Michigan experiments (5) more cases of necrotic enteritis developed on the basal ration of corn than when barley was fed. Supplementing the corn ration with fresh liver (200 grams daily), yeast or liver meal instead of tankage, or changing the grain ration to barley often resulted in curing the condition. It was also found that it was necessary to give as much as 100 to 300 milligrams of nicotinic acid a day in order to prevent or cure the symptoms of necrotic enteritis which were attributed to nicotinic acid deficiency. Successful use of nicotinic acid to treat this condition in swine under farm conditions was reported by the Michigan workers and also by Madison and co-workers (23) at the Pennsylvania station.

Because of the widespread losses of pigs due to necrotic enteritis and similar conditions, more work needs to be done to define the relationships of diet and infection as causes of this disease more accurately, as well as to obtain additional information on the content of protective factors in available swine feeds.

Pyridoxine (Vitamin B_6) Deficiency

Chick and associates (4) fed young swine on a purified diet and noted that the animals developed typical epileptic fits and a microcytic anemia (characterized by small red blood corpuscles) if they were deprived of the fraction of yeast containing vitamin B_6. Van Etten, Ellis, and Madsen (*27*), in studies on the thiamin requirement of swine, noted convulsions in swine fed autoclaved (heated) diets, and in later studies of the Bureau of Animal Industry, convulsions and anemia were found to occur in young pigs on both autoclaved and synthetic diets which did not contain crystalline pyridoxine. This deficiency is not apt to occur under farm conditions unless the swine are fed a restricted diet low in this factor or unless the vitamin has been destroyed by unusual treatment of the ration.

Pyridoxine is of little interest at this time in livestock-feeding because of its wide distribution in natural foods, including the cereal grains and legumes. Yeast and glandular tissue such as kidney and liver are also good sources. This factor is synthesized by bacteria in the digestive tract of ruminants but must be present in the diets of chickens, dogs, and swine.

Pantothenic Acid Deficiency

Pantothenic acid was first recognized as a growth-promoting factor in yeast. It has now been established as an essential vitamin for several species of animals. Dry-heat treatment of feed readily destroys the factor. Bacteria synthesize this vitamin in the digestive tracts of ruminants, but chickens, dogs, swine, and possibly some other animals require the factor preformed in the diet. Experiments in feeding purified and heat-treated rations at the Beltsville Research Centre indicate that young swine on rations deficient in this factor lose their appetite, grow slowly or stop gaining in weight for a time, then lose weight and die (Fig. 6). Other prominent symptoms of this deficiency are diarrhoea (frequently bloody), loss of hair, weakness and incoordination in the use of the legs, and the formation of a brownish-red incrusted material on the eyelids. Microscopic examination of the nerves and spinal cords from pantothenic-acid-deficient pigs has revealed degeneration of the myelin (sheath) of the nerve fibers similar in all details to that found in pigs that developed incoordination on natural feeds and heat-treated rations (*6*), as described in the following section of this article.

Hughes (*17*) and Hughes and Ittner (*18*) have also studied pantothenic acid deficiency in swine, and they suggest that the minimum requirement for this factor fed as calcium pantothenate

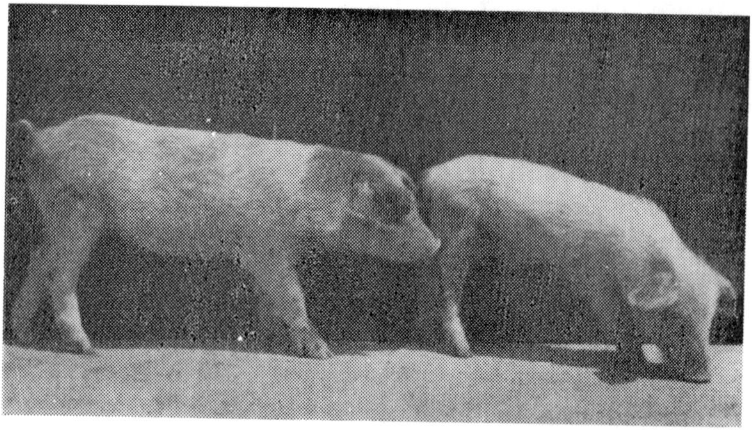

Fig. 6: Both these pigs were fed the same purified diet except that the pig on the right did not get a supplement of pantothenic acid. This animal has a poor appetite, is weak and emaciated, and suffers from severe diarrhoea.

lies between 7.8 and 11.8 milligrams daily for each 100 pounds of live weight.

Locomotor Incoordination in Swine Due to Nerve Degeneration

A varying number of pigs fed in pens on rations that have heretofore been considered nutritionally complete–such as yellow corn and trio protein mixture (tankage, linseed meal, and alfalfa), with a supplementary mineral mixture–develop incoordination in the use of their legs. This disease was probably first described by Wehrbein in 1916 at the Iowa State College as posterior paralysis and incoordination in movement, associated with degeneration of the sheath of various nerves. Communications to the Bureau of Animal Industry indicate that the disorder is of serious economic importance and is more prevalent during some years than others. It has occurred in the Bureau's herd at the Beltsville Research Centre, Beltsville, Md.

Recent work on the problem by Ellis and Madsen (6) has shown that feeding normal diets that have been subjected for 30 to 40 hours to dry heat at a temperature of 115°-120° F. greatly increases the

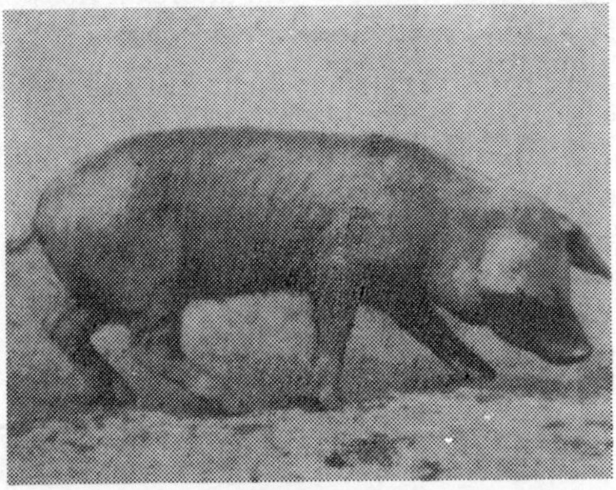

Fig. 7: This pig has marked incoordination in the use of its legs owing to nerve degeneration. The incidence and severity of the disease can be increased by heating the ration.

incidence of the disease and the severity of myelin degeneration in the nerves and spinal cord (Fig. 7). Supplemental or replacement feeds fed with the heated diet have given some encouraging results. Barley, oats, liver, and concentrated milk products have given the most protection. Tests with many other feeds plainly indicate that the dietary factor or factors involved are present in variable or insufficient amounts in many of the common swine feeds. Further work with purified and natural-food diets at the Beltsville Research Centre, together with the work of Wintrobe and associates (*30*) and the recent report by Hughes (*17*), indicates that pantothenic acid deficiency is probably one of the causes if not the main cause of this disease.

Acute Hypoglycemia in Newborn Pigs, or so-called Baby Pig Disease

For a number of years the Illinois Agricultural Experiment Station has been investigating a highly fatal disease of newborn pigs. Sampson, Hester, and Graham (*26*) describe the symptoms of this condition as follows:

In the typical syndrome apparently normal pigs varying from approximately 24 hours to 72 hours old or slightly older show symptoms of shivering, dullness, and anorexia (loss of appetite). The animals have a tendency to isolate themselves and burrow under the bedding. * * * Coincident with the loss of appetite and onset of weakness, the hair coat becomes rough, the skin cold and clammy, and the heart action slow and feeble. Finally the pig lapses into coma. Death of several or all pigs in the litter often occurs within 24 to 36 hours after the first symptoms are manifested.

These investigators report that the affected animals have a maked lowering of the blood sugar, or hypoglycemia, and indicate that the symptoms are probably due to this feature of the disease. In experimental work, baby pigs were found to be highly susceptible to a lowered blood sugar caused by fasting up to about 24 hours after birth. Affected pigs have been successfully treated in the early stages of the disease by repeated intraperitoneal injections of glucose supplemented by hand feeding of sugar solution or milk. Suggested preventive measures include feeding sows and gilts a liberal ration throughout pregnancy and not reducing the amount of grain fed during the last few weeks of the gestation period as commonly practiced. New-born pigs should be closely watched for the first few days to be sure that they are nursing properly, that the sow has sufficient milk, and that the young pigs do not become chilled. If symptoms develop, hand feeding should be begun immediately.

Literature Cited

(1) AUBEL, E.C., HUGHES, J.S., and LEINHARIDT, H.F. (1936). THE EFFECTS OF LOW-PHOSPHORUS RATIONS ON GROWING PIGS. Jour. Agr. Res. 52: 149-159, illus.

(2) BETHKE, R.M., EDGINGTON, B.H., and KICK, C.H. (1933). EFFECT OF THE CALCIUM-PHOSPHORUS RELATIONSHIP OF THE RATION ON GROWTH AND BONE FORMATION IN THE PIG. Jour. Agr. Res. 47: 331-338, illus.

(3) CHICK, HARRIETTE; MACRAE, THOMAS FOTHERINGHAM; MARTIN, ARCHER JOHN PORTER; and MARTIN, CHARLES JAMES (1938). CURATIVE ACTION OF NICOTINIC ACID ON PIGS SUFFERING FROM THE EFFECTS OF A DIET CONSISTING LARGELY OF MAIZE. Biochem. Jour. 32(1): 10-12, illus.

(4) _____MACRAE, THOMAS FOTHERINGHAM; MARTIN, ARCHER JOHN PORTER; and MARTIN, CHARLES JAMES (1938). THE WATER-SOLUBLE B-VITAMINS OTHER THAN ANEURIN (VITAMIN B_1), RIBOFLAVIN AND NICOTINIC ACID REQUIRED BY THE PIG. Biochem. Jour. 32 (3): 2207-2224, illus.

(5) DAVIS, G.K., FREEMAN, V.A. and MADSEN, L.L. (1940). THE RELATION OF NUTRITION TO THE DEVELOPMENT OF NECROTIC ENTERITIS IN SWINE. Mich. Agr. Expt. Sta. Tech. Bul. 170, 23 pp., illus.

(6) ELLIS, N.R., and MADSEN, L.L. (1941). RELATION OF DIET OF SWINE TO DEVELOPMENT OF LOCOMOTOR INCORDINATION RESULTING FROM NERVE DEGENERATION. Jour. Agr. Res. 62: 303-316, illus.

(7) _____and ZELLER, J.H. (1939). NUTRITIVE REQUIREMENTS OF SWINE. U.S. Dept. Agr. Yearbook (Food and Life) 1939: 706-722, illus.

(8) EVANS, R.E. (1929). PROTEIN AND MINERAL METABOLISM IN PREGNANT BOWS ON A NORMAL OR HIGH CALCIUM DIET COMPARED WITH A CALCIUM-DEFICIENT DIET. Jour. Agr. Sci. [England] 19: 752-798, illus.

(9) GARDNER, V.R. (1938). NECROTIC ENTERITIS IN SWINE. (Preliminary note) Mich. Agr. Expt. Sta. Rpt. 1937-38: 14.

(10) GUILBERT, H.R., MILLER, R.F., and HUGHES, E.H. (1937). THE MINIMUM VITAMIN A AND CAROTENE REQUIREMENT OF CATTLE, SHEEP AND SWINE. Jour. Nutr. 13: 543-564.

(11) HALE, FRED (1935). THE RELATION OF VITAMIN A TO ANOPHTHALMOS IN PIGS. Amer. Jour. Ophth. 18: 1087-1092, illus.

(12) HOGAN, A.G. (1932). THE CALCIUM REQUIREMENT OF BROOD SOWS. Mo. Agr. Expt. Sta. Res. Bul. 167, 18 pp., illus.

(13) HOSTETLER, EARL H., FOSTER, J.E., and HALVERSON, J.O. (1935). VITAMIN A DEFICIENCY–A CAUSE OF LAMENESS AND DEATH AMONG SWINE. N.C. Agr. Expt. Sta. Tech. Bul. 52, 31 pp., illus.

(14) HUGHES, E.H. (1938). THE VITAMIN-B COMPLEX AS RELATED TO GROWTH AND METABOLISM IN THE PIG. Hilgardia 11: 593-612, illus.

(15) _____(1939). THE ROLE OF RIBOFLAVIN AND OTHER FACTORS OF THE VITAMIN-B COMPLEX IN THE NUTRITION OF THE PIG. Jour. Nutr. 17: 527-533, illus.

(16) _____(1940). THE MINIMUM REQUIREMENT OF RIBOFLAVIN FOR THE GROWING PIG. Jour. Nutr. 20: 233-238; illus.

(17) _____(1942). PANTOTHENIC ACID IN THE NUTRITION OF THE PIG. Jour. Agr. Res. 64: 185-187, illus.

(18) HUGHES, E.H., and ITTNER, N.R. (1942). THE MINIMUM REQUIREMENT OF PANTOTHENIC ACID FOR THE GROWING PIG. (Abstract of paper) Jour. Anim. Sci. 1: 85.

(19) HUGHES, J.S., AUBEL, A.E., and LIENHARDT, H.F. (1928). THE IMPORTANCE OF VITAMIN A AND VITAMIN IN THE RATION OF SWINE, CONCERNING ESPECIALLY THEIR EFFECT ON GROWTH AND REPRODUCTION. Kans. Agr. Expt. Sta. Tech. Bul. 23, 48 pp., illus.

(20) JOHNSON, D.W., and PALMER, L.S. (1939). INDIVIDUAL AND BREED VARIATIONS IN PIGS ON RATIONS DEVOID OF VITAMIN D. Jour. Agr. Res. 58: 929-940.

(21) KICK, C.H., BETHKE, R.M., and EDGINGTON, B.H. (1933). EFFECT OF FLUORINE ON THE NUTRITION OF SWINE, WITH SPECIAL REFERENCE TO BONE AND TOOTH COMPOSITION. Jour. Agr. Res. 46: 1023-1037, illus.

(22) LOEFFEL, WM.J., THALMAN, RAY R., OLSON, F.C. and OLSON, F.A. (1931). STUDIES OF RICKETS IN SWINE. Nebr. Agr. Expt. Sta. Res. Bul. 58, 67 pp., illus.

(23) MADISON, L.C., MILLER, R.C., and KEITH, T.B. (1939). NICOTINIC ACID IN SWINE NUTRITION. Science 89: 490-491.

(24) MILLER, R.C., KEITH, T.B., McCARTHY, M.A., and THORP, W.T.S. (1940). MANGANESE AS A POSSIBLE FACTOR INFLUENCING THE OCCURRENCE OF LAMENESS IN PIGS. Soc. Expt. Biol. and Med. Proc. 45: 50-51.

(25) MOXON, ALVIN L. (1937). ALKALI DISEASE OR SELENIUM POISONING. S. Dak. Agr. Expt. Sta. Bul. 311, 91 pp., illus.

(26) SAMPSON, JESSE, HESTER, H.R., and GRAHAM, ROBERT (1942). STUDIES ON BABY-PIG MORTALITY. II. FURTHER OBSERVATIONS ON ACUTE HYPOGLYCEMIA IN NEWLY BORN PIGS (SO-CALLED BABY-PIG, DISEASE). Amer. Vet. Med. Assoc. Jour. 100: 33-37, illus.

(27) VAN ETTEN, CECIL, ELLIS, N.R., and MADSEN, L.L. (1940). STUDIES ON THE THIAMIN REQUIREMENT OF YOUNG SWINE. Jour. Nutr. 20: 607-625, illus.

(28) WELCH, HOWARD (1940). PREVENTION OF GOITER ON FARM ANIMALS. Mont. Agr. Expt. Sta. Cir. 160, 5 pp., illus.

(29) WILLMAN, J.P., McCAY, C.M., and MORRISON, F.B. (1932). ANEMIA IN SUCKLING PIGS. Amer. Soc. Anim. Prod. Proc. 25: 141-145.

(30) WINTROBE, MAXWELL W., MITCHELL, DAVID M., and KOLB, LAWRENCE C. (1938). SENSORY NEURON DEGENERATION IN VITAMIN DEFICIENCY. DEGENERATION OF THE POSTERIOR COLUMNS OF THE SPINAL CORD, PERIPHERAL NERVES, AND DORSAL ROOT GANGLION CELLS IN YOUNG PIGS FED A DIET CONTAINING THIAMIN (B_1) AND RIBOFLAVIN BUT OTHERWISE DEFICIENT IN VITAMIN B COMPLEX. Jour. Expt. Med. 68: 207-220, illus.

(31) ZELLER, J.H., and ELLIS, N.R. (1939). PRACTICES IN SWINE FEEDING. U.S. Dept. Agr. Yearbook (Food and Life) 1939: 723-745, illus.

INDEX

A

Arthritis, 48

Ascaris lumbricoides, 140

B

Babcock, O.G., 107

Bacillus murisepticus, 37

B. suipestifier, 50

Bacterium choleraesuis, 50

Balantidium coli, 145

Brucella abortus, 92

Brucella melitensis, 93

Brucella organism, 9

Brucella suis, 9, 95, 96

Brucellosis (infectious abortion) in swine
- diagnosis, 95
- lesions, 93-94
- prevention and control, 95-96
- public health hazard, 96-97
- symptoms, 94-95

Brucellosis (infectious abortion) of swine, 9
- bang's disease organism of cattle, 9

Bureau of Animal Industry, 23, 61, 183

C

Choerostrongylus pudendotectus, 129

Control measures
- anti-swine-erysipelas serum, 46
- crude petroleum, 109
- immunization, 46, 55
- serum-and-culture method of vaccination, 46

Creech, G.T., 6, 73

Crystal-violet vaccine
- anti-hog-cholera serum, 36
- vaccine, 36

Cushing, E.C., 107

D

Dale, C.N., 4, 5, 49, 59

Diseases of swine, 1, 6, 73

E

Echinococcus granulosus, 117

Eichhorn, Adolph., 92

Ellis, N.R., 18, 187

Endamoeba, 144

Endolimax, 144

Enteritis of swine, 4, 49
- casual organism, 50-51

cause and lesions, 55-56
control measures, 52-53, 56-57
enteritis and scours in baby pigs, 57-58
due to miscellaneous causes, 58
lesions, 51-52
necrotic enteritis, 49-50
relation of nutrition to necrotic enteritis, 53
swine dysentery, 53-54
symptoms, 51, 54-55

Erysipelothrix rhusiopathiae, 38, 41

F

Fasciola hepatica, 118
Flu, 60
Flukes, 114

G

Grey, C.G., 2, 37

H

Hemophilus influenzae suis, 59,, 62-66, 68
Hog cholera, 21, 47
anti-hog cholera serum, 31-35
cause of hog cholera, 23
crystal-violet vaccine, 35-36
economic losses, 21
immunization, 33
importance of sanitation and care in the prevention of disease, 30-31
modes of infection, 28-30
monetary value of hogs destroyed by cholera, 21
post mortem findings, 26-28
prevention, 31
seasonal occurrence, 25-26
symptoms and diagnosis, 23-25
virus, 51
Hog flu, 24
lice, 10, 102, 107
control measures, 109-110
dipping and treating, 110-111
how hog lice breed, 108
Hog-cholera virus, 55
Hyostrongylus rubidus, 120

I

Imes, Marion, 98
Internal parasites of swine, 11, 112
amoebae, 144-145
balantidia, 145-146
coccidia, 147
control by management, 150
treatment, 148-149
kidney worms, 131-136
hook worms, 137
thorn-headed worms, 137-140
McLean county system of swine sanitation, 150-151
advantages obtained by use of the system, 155-158
kidney worm control plan, 158-163
procedures under the system, 151-155
result obtained by use of the system, 163-165
protozoan parasites, 144
sarcocystis, 148
thorn-headed worms.
large intestinal roundworms (ascarids), 140-144

worm parasites, 116
flukes, 118
gullet worms, 119-120
hydatid, 117-118
intestinal threadworms, 122-124
lungworms, 129-131
nodular worms, 124-127
pork bladder worm, 116-117
roundworms, 118-119
stomach worms, 120-122
tapeworms, 116
thin-necked bladder worm, 118
whipworms, 127-129

Iodamoeba, 144

K

Kidney worms
loin muscles, 135
control of kidney worms, 162
ureters, 134

Kidneys, 134

L

Large intestinal roundworms (ascarids): roundworms, 141
Larvae of June bugs, 138
Lice, 107, 108, 109
Liver destruction, 134

M

Macrocanthorhynchus hirudinaceus, 137
Madsen, Louis L., 18, 20, 196
Mange of swine, 10, 98
contagiousness, 101-102
demodectic mange, 105-1096
sarcoptic mange, 99-100
symptoms, 100-101
treatment, 102-103
dips, 103-104
methods of applying dips, 104-105
May beetles, 138
McBryde, C.N., 1, 21
McLean County system of sanitation, 14, 150
Metastrongylus elongatus, 129
M. salmi, 129
Miscellaneous diseases of swine, 6, 73
diagnosis and control measures, 76, 90-91
diagnosis, treatment and prevention, 76
eczema, 87-88
erythema, 86-87
goiter (hairless pigs), 7, 80-82
infectious arthritis, 7, 76-78
mastitis (mammitis, or garget), 84-86
mastitis, 8
necrotic rhinitis, 7, 78-80
paralysis of the hindquarters, 7
pneumonia, 7, 82-84
skin diseases of swine, 86
stomatitis, 7, 78-80
sunburn and frostbite, 88
swine plague (hemorrhagic septicemia), 89-90
swine pox, 73-76
urticaria (nettle rash), 87
Mouse neutralization tests, 67
septicemia bacillus, 37

N

National Institute for Medical Research, London, 65
Necrotic enteritis, 49, 51, 52

acid deficiency and necrotic enteritis in swine: swine feeds, 212
Nutritional diseases of swine, 18, 196
control of, 196
iodine deficiency and the birth of weak pigs, 204-205
mineral deficiency diseases of swine, 197
cause, prevention, and treatment, 198-200
rickets, 199
calcium deficiency in brood sows, 200-201
phosphorus deficiency, 202
rickets, 197-198
nutritional anemia of suckling pigs, 202-204
toxic minerals, 205
fluorine and selenium poisoning, 205
vitamin deficiency diseases of swine, 205
acute hypoglycemia in newborn pigs, or so-called baby pig disease, 215-216
locomotor incoordination in swine due to nerve degeneration, 214-215
nicotinic acid deficiency and necrotic enteritis in swine, 211-212
pantothenic acid deficiency, 213-214
pyridoxine (vitamin B6) deficiency, 212-213
riboflavin deficiency, 210-211
thiamin (vitamin B1) deficiency, 209-210
vitamin A deficiency, 205-209

O

Oesophagostomum brevicaudum, 124, 125
O. dentatum, 124, 125, 127
O. georgianum, 124
O. longicaudum, 124, 125, 126
Osteen, O.L., 2, 37

P

Paragonimus westermanii, 118
Permanent pastures perpetuate parasites, 115
Physocephalus sexalatus, 121
Pigs, 62, 63, 112, 120, 123, 127, 150, 165, 191, 193, 194
affected with swine influenza, 62
Protozoa, 114

R

Relation to arthritis, 46
Roundworms, 114

S

Salmonella choleraesuis, 49, 50, 51, 53, 54, 55
S. suipestifer, 50
Salt tolerance and salt poisoning of swine, 18, 187-193
Sarcocystis miescheriana, 148
Schoening, H.W., 2, 237
Schwartz, Beniamin, 16, 17, 167
Sick animals, 5
Skin diseases, 8
eczema, 8
erythema, 8
freezing, or frostbite, 8-9
sunburn, 8
urticaria, 8
Spindler, L.A., 11, 14, 15, 112
Stephanurus dentatus, 131

Strongyloides ransomi, 122
Swine cholera *Salmonella*, 50
- erysipelas, 2, 3, 37, 44, 45, 48
- control measures, 45-46
- diagnosis, 44-45
- differential diagnosis, 47-48
- nature and cause of the disease, 38-41
- relation to arthritis, 46-47
- symptoms, 41-44
- influenza, 5, 59, 60, 61, 63, 69
- action of the human influenza virus in swine, 68-69
- cause of human influenza determines, 65
- comparative studies of swine and human viruses, 66-68
- experiments that lead to finding the cause of swine influenza, 62-64
- immunity experiments, 64-65
- lung, 67
- other recent findings, 69-70
- parasites, control, 148-150
- plague, 9
- raiser, 115
- research on swine and human influenza, 60-61
- virus, 70

Symptoms
- anti-hog-cholera, 51
- serum for immunization, 55

T

Taenia hydatigena, 118
Tapeworms, 114
Traum's discovery of brucellosis in swine, 93
Trichina-infected meat, 170
Trichinella spiralis, 167, 168, 171
Trichinosis, 16, 167
Trichuris suis, 127
Types of influenza, 70

U

United States Bureau of Entomology and Plant Quarantine, 29-30

W

White grubs, 138